SEX IS NEVER AN EMERGENCY

MUTUALLY DESIRED SEXUAL ACTIVITY IS NEVER SUCH AN EMERGENCY THAT PREGNANCY CANNOT BE AVOIDED, EVEN IF IT IS NECESSARY TO SUBSTITUTE, TEMPORARILY, ONE OF THE VERY SATISFACTORY VARIATIONS OF ABSTINENCE.

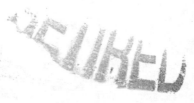

THIRD EDITION

SEX IS NEVER AN EMERGENCY

A Candid Guide for Young Adults

Elaine C. Pierson, Ph.D., M.D.
(Mrs. Luigi Mastroianni, Jr.)

J. B. LIPPINCOTT COMPANY

Philadelphia • New York • Toronto

First edition. Copyright © 1970 by Elaine C. Pierson.
Second edition. Copyright © 1971 by Elaine C. Pierson.
Third edition. Copyright © 1973 by Elaine C. Pierson.

ISBN 0-397-47291-9

Library of Congress Catalog Card Number 78-148244

1 3 5 7 9 8 6 4 2

PRINTED IN THE UNITED STATES OF AMERICA

Pierson, Elaine Catherine
    Sex is never an emergency.

    First ed. published in 1970 under title:
A guide for University of Pennsylvania
students, 1970–71.
    Bibliography: p.
    1. Sex instruction for youth.
2. Conception––Prevention. 3. College
students––Sexual behavior. I. Title.
[DNLM: 1. Contraception––Popular works.
2. Sex manuals. HQ31 P624s 1973]
HQ35.2.P53 1973   301.41'75   78-148244
ISBN 0-397-47292-7
ISBN 0-397-47291-9 (pbk.)

Contents

156197

Preface to the Third Edition

Our primary objective for this third edition remains the same as in earlier editions: prevention of accidental pregnancies. However, growing public awareness of the need for this kind of information now permits discussion of a number of related areas without jeopardizing general acceptance. There have been modifications of some contraceptive methods, but very little change in the basic ones. There has also been a growing willingness among students and young adults to ask questions, to admit their lack of knowledge about physiology and function, and to do some "prospective" rather than retrospective thinking about sexual activity. Prospective thinking must include an awareness that *for females* as well as males there is a "point of no return" during sexual stimulation—the real endpoint of seduction—when the words "No" or "Not now" suddenly and briefly disappear from one's vocabulary.

Much of the material in this book appeared originally in article form in the *Daily Pennsylvanian*. It was written in response to questions about contraceptives and related areas, mostly from male students, and is the result of five years at the University of Pennsylvania doing office gynecology in the student health service, and talking to girls, on request, about contraceptives as well as seeing students from other colleges and universities in the Philadelphia area at a Planned Parenthood clinic. It is also the result of our association, direct and *indirect*, with student populations in five major universities over the past 30 years, and our having lived with obstetrics and gynecology, figuratively and literally, for the past 16 years.

The revisions in this edition are minor. New material has been added in the sections on abortion and the Pill that reflects the current thinking on these subjects. Additional questions and answers have been included in response to requests by students and young adults. But the basic philosophy remains unchanged — old-fashioned puritan ethics. We like to think that it represents the puritan ethic as Norman Mailer once defined it, "*Pragmatism without hypocrisy.*"

We have also continued to use the nonjudgmental approach, although we dislike this and feel that it denotes either laziness or fear of criticism. But given our primary objective and wanting to reach the maximum audience we are convinced that it is the only approach to use. It does not necessarily imply that we approve of the gestalt of the sixties and seventies that created the problem. And although it is very difficult to answer some questions (all real questions) without sounding like a militant feminist, we can only say that we are not militant, except in one or two specific areas.

It has become apparent with the new openness that there are many questions about the external anatomy of males and females, not to mention the internal anatomy. We have thus added for this edition some drawings which were designed to be more than outlines and less than photographs. Drawings and photographs of the average adult female perineum have been available for thousands of years, but with the exception of gross pornography, reproductions of normal, circumcized, adult male genitals have been very difficult to find, even in anatomy texts and medical books. When they do appear in medical texts they are always pictured with disease or not attached to a body, or simply as isolated pieces of anatomy. This is our small contribution to the cause of antimale chauvinism.

We have continued to avoid percentages in describing the effectiveness of any contraceptive method. All methods can be and are misused, including the Pill, with resultant pregnancies. There continue to be only high risk or low risk methods, and none can be considered 100 percent effective in actual usage, even for the well motivated.

We have also kept the book short and concise, though we could do twenty pages on the diaphragm alone.

However, we know from experience that much of this information will only be read when the need for it arises, often, we have found, after the fact, and that young people often need verbal reassurance of anything they read about sexual activity. In the absence of sexual activity involving the genital area, this kind of information is always of importance "to someone else." In the presence of good sexual activity, further information is often "unnecessary" since everything is working as well as can be expected.

We believe in allowing the slow evolution of one's sexuality–it doesn't "all" happen the first time or every time, routinely. But there are often questions that need answers now, and verbal assurance is not always available.

Elaine C. Pierson, Ph.D., M.D.
(Mrs. Luigi Mastroianni, Jr.)

Philadelphia
September 1973

Introduction

This guide was written to give young adults a basic understanding of the physical and emotional aspects of contraception and to provide information about the related areas of sexual performance, hygiene, and disease. We hope that this information will relieve some of the anxiety which can result from involvement or the thought of eventual involvement in the physical aspects of sexuality. A little anxiety is a good thing. It keeps people on their toes and makes life interesting. But the male-female relationship is complicated enough without being hampered by additional concerns arising from ignorance or lack of knowledge about the pure mechanics of the relationship.

We have provided enough information to help both of you—males and females—stay out of trouble. The most devastating trouble, as defined by young adults and their parents, is the unwanted pregnancy. Neither of you wants a pregnancy now. You may consider abortion to be the ultimate contraceptive, but abortion is not a benign procedure, even when done under ideal conditions (see Complications, p. 34). In many instances, the impact of abortion is felt by both of the individuals involved. Men may feel the responsibility for the risk of abortion more intensely than women because they are relatively helpless in the situation. They can offer only emotional or financial support, knowing that neither can really be equated with the risk. They may not even have the opportunity to do this because, as those who have been confronted by a girl seriously intent on abortion know, she may brush everyone and everything aside, including *his* emotional support and money, unless there is a desperate need for the latter. The risk of abortion is "low on her list." Who, When, and Where are her only concerns.

Nor is a hasty marriage benign. A wife and child, or a husband and child, will redirect your whole life, at a time when you both thought you still had some options. To continue your life as before is impossible, even if it is a good marriage.

For the girl, carrying a pregnancy to term and delivering the child to its adopting parents is not benign, although it is probably better for her uterus than a late abortion. Raising an unplanned child without a father might be fun for the first nine months, but then babies cease being toys. The girl who is "keeping" the pregnancy should ask herself two questions: 1) Am I keeping it because I need the child or because the child needs me? 2) Would I feel differently about raising a boy vs. raising a girl?

In the face of pregnancy, a single girl has only four options: marriage, or in the absence of a male, raising the child, giving the child away, or having an abortion. None of these is particularly attractive.

DO NOT FIGHT CONTRACEPTION. It is a way of life for most responsible people. Your sexual activity should be considered realistically within its limits. *Contraception must also be a mutual responsibility.* Men should know as much about rhythm, withdrawal, diaphragms, and so on as women. You both have over 30 years of contraception ahead of you, and you both should begin to understand early that the physical aspects of sexuality can be very good, even within this limitation.

For Virgins: Male and Female

Do not apologize to yourself or anyone else. You may be part of an apolitical silent majority—that large, discreet group that doesn't talk about the extent or level of its sexual activities—at least for the present. Premarital sexual activity has almost as many reasons for existing as there are individuals involved, and the reasons are not all negative. Nor does it have to be a totally negative experience; you can learn from all experiences.

The inability to form good interpersonal relationships

with a variety of people of both sexes may often be the basis for a desperate one-to-one relationship over a long or short term. This may offer just the right amount of security that will allow an individual to function in other areas. It may also create unanticipated problems.

Some young adults form good relationships easily, with or without overt sexuality. Such relationships may be good sexually or only superficially good, with a large element of sexual hostility. This hostility may take many forms, from abstinence to gross promiscuity. Hostility directed toward parents or toward oneself can take the form of obvious sexual activity, male or female, carried to the point of the "accidental" pregnancy.

Some young adults are unable to handle the freedom of dormitory living. They cannot say "my parents" or "that Dean" or "that dorm says I have to be in by 11 P.M." They have to make their own decisions. There is no nest. Some solve this problem by creating a nest, which provides someone who cares where they are and what they are doing.

You may be faced, as your parents were, with rather compelling arguments: "How can we really know each other unless we 'know' each other?" or "A marriage license should mean more than a license to have intercourse. Don't you agree? What are you saving yourself for?" Be aware that there is increasing respect for individual choice, and options are becoming more available so that you can make a choice without being forced into one pattern or another. If you sincerely believe in being your own self, "virgin" is not a bad word, whether applied to males or females. This still takes some courage, however, so perhaps the easiest way for a few more years is just to keep quiet about your sexual life. Decisions about heavy petting presented similar difficult problems for some of your parents, just as intercourse does for many young people today—but no pregnancies were involved in that variation of abstinence.

Consider these points when you look around and

think that something is wrong with you. Self-analysis, or analysis with help, need not change your mind or your feelings, but at least you will be in a better position to learn from your observation of others and, more important, not get hurt or hurt another person.

Legal Aspects of Medical Care

It is important that you know about the legal aspects of medical care in your state and the laws regarding minors and medical care of any kind, including pregnancy, venereal disease, and other reportable diseases. You should also know about the abortion law and whether or not the individual who has had an *illegal abortion* is criminally liable.

Please note that with respect to medical care, regardless of the law, there is nothing that says a physician must treat you, whether or not parental consent is necessary. Also, even in states with liberal laws about minors and medical care, the laws are variously construed and often do not include abortion without parental consent, even though they state that pregnancy in a minor may be treated. And even disreputable physicians will not accede to requests from 18-year-olds for tubal ligations and vasectomies, unless there are clear genetic (hereditary) or medical reasons, and these are few and far between.

Methods of Contraception

Realistically, the only truly "safe" methods are the nonvaginal variations of abstinence, vas and tubal ligation, condoms, pills, diaphragm with gel, the IUD, and that part of the menstrual cycle three days after there has been a rise in the basal body temperature. The remaining methods are either at the research level or less than adequate. Percentage effectiveness is of little value; there are only high risk and low risk methods. Even the pill is often so grossly misused that it cannot be called 100 percent effective in any large population, as this will include all poorly motivated, or uninformed users.

METHODS OF CONTRACEPTION CURRENTLY AVAILABLE

Male and Female	Male	Female
ABSTINENCE	WITHDRAWAL	SPERMICIDES†
total	CONDOMS	foam, cream, gels
periodic	VASECTOMY*	diaphragm with
rhythm		OVULATION PREVENTION**
basal body		oral
temperature (BBT)		injectable
nonvaginal variations		implanted
masturbation		UNKNOWN ACTION
solitary		minipill
mutual		morning after pill
oralgenital		intrauterine device
anal intercourse		mechanical
		chemical
		hormonal
		heavy metals (copper)

TUBAL STERILIZATION

* See References, "Contraceptive Research: A Male Chauvinist Plot?"
† Douching is not a contraceptive method.

** Breast-feeding is not a contraceptive method.
# Abortion is not a contraceptive method.

Withdrawal

QUESTION: If withdrawal is complete before ejaculation, is it a safe method of contraception?

ANSWER: Withdrawal or coitus interruptus is just that, interrupted intercourse. It leaves a great deal to be desired both in satisfaction and safety. Many couples use it routinely, but if you consider the points below you will realize that it cannot approach 100 percent effectiveness, although actual percentages are difficult to obtain for obvious reasons.

1. It requires skill as a result of much practice, willpower, and the necessity for awareness on the part of the male at a time when emotions may overshadow rational thought.

2. There is only a period of about three to five seconds from the time the male is aware of the inevitability of ejaculation to acual ejaculation.

3. There is a preejaculatory secretion ranging in quantity from a few drops to as much as 1 cc. of seminal fluid. This is especially true when erection is prolonged. This fluid frequently has motile sperm in it, and we must assume that they are capable of fertilizing an egg.

4. Ejaculation in the introital area (hymeneal, vaginal opening) in the presence of normal vaginal secretions puts sperm in the position to migrate to the cervix. Most gynecologists have heard histories from pregnant patients that would confirm this as a remote possibility.

5. At best, withdrawal as a method of contraception is a compromise. It requires a tremendous amount of concentration and willpower on the part of the male and trust on the part of the female. This trust is not always well founded and creates anxiety. Neither factor is conducive to relaxatio.. and pleasure, and both leave the couple with a very distorted idea of what it is all about.

Condoms

Questions and Comments from a student (male) discussion about condoms as a contraceptive:

QUESTIONS

Are they safe? Yes, if used properly. Proper use means: 1) using it prior to any approach to entry to catch that pre-ejaculatory secretion which may contain active sperm, 2) leaving room at end for the ejaculate, and   3) holding the condom when withdrawing. Withdrawal should occur before complete loss of erection or the condom may be left behind.

Do they break often? No, if you avoid the fifteen and twenty-cent brands. "The condom broke" is usually what the couple says when they come for help after a failed withdrawal. There are two situations in which a condom might break: 1) if you fumble when you try to apply it initially and attempt to use the same one again (carry more than one), 2) if decreased vaginal lubrication makes penetration difficult. Occasionally there may be an indication for the lubricated condom but this is generally unpleasant to use (initially cold and may cause a stinging sensation in a sensitive vagina), as well as being more expensive. To solve the former problem, ask the druggist for a surgical lubricant such as K-Y jelly. Vaseline is impossible.

Does the condom prevent VD? Probably, if unprotected contact is avoided, although this is not usually the way condoms are used. They are usually used at the last possible moment, after external genital or intravaginal contact has occurred. If used properly, they would theoretically be more effective in preventing the male from acquiring gonorrhea from an infected female than vice-versa, because any unprotected, initial, external genital contact with the infected female is less likely to transmit gonorrhea to the male than is intravaginal contact. The unprotected, infected male can transmit gonorrhea or syphilis to the female genital or oral area easily with any kind of penile contact. Condoms protect against infection and reinfection by the Trichomonas organism which is relatively common in females. This is asymptomatic in males but causes an uncomfortable, vaginal discharge in the female that requires medical treatment. Occasionally, when reinfection occurs in the female, the male must be treated also.

Condoms may protect the male from a nonspecific urethritis (NSU) discussed later (see VD). The advent of the pill and the availability of the diaphragm have led to a decline in the use of condoms which may be contributing to an apparent increase in this type of urethritis in the male. However, NSU is not necessarily related, in all instances, to sexual activity.

COMMENTS

Condoms allow me to be in control. True, and everyone likes to be in control.* Also, there are some casual or even some long-term relationships which cannot be trusted. Is the girl really on the pill? Is she using the diaphragm properly? Does she want to get pregnant? A small percentage of girls are not conscious of their desire to get pregnant but simply think that they are "taking a chance," just this once. It is a poor way to get even with their families, or with you, or to get a man, but it happens.

Condoms decrease sensation. True. But who has the claim on sensation? You or the girl who pops a pill in her mouth every day and reads the almost daily antipill reports, and wonders what she is doing to herself? She is sensitive every day, not just for an occasional few minutes, to the side effects of the pill, even if they are only the recurrent yeast overgrowths which plague many girls. Many relate every little twinge or symptom they have, leg ache, breast soreness, a small blue vein, and so on, to the pill they are taking. This sounds like a feminist argument, but it is simply a plea from one who has seen many girls and can appreciate their problems, not to push the pill on someone in a threatening way. There is an implicit threat when she is asked to take the pill for her complexion problems. There is a very real

---

* It is possible that condoms decrease sensation just enough to prolong the pleasure (erection) prior to ejaculation (see Premature Ejaculation).

threat when he says that he is absolutely not going to use a condom and that he doesn't want to see her fussing around with a diaphragm. We are not antipill, but many married and unmarried women, who are uncomfortable with the emotional and physical aspects of the pill, are taking it anyway because someone they really care about would like them to use it.

Condoms don't give me total freedom. True, but there is nothing like a baby, yours, or a pregnant girl friend to impress you with what freedom really is. Are girls *free* who take a pill every day so they may be available once or twice a week, or who carry a diaphragm at all times, just in case? Or those who are feeling for the strings of the IUD every other day, or worrying about every mild uterine cramp, and wondering if they should be using foam with their IUD to be really safe? Who has the claim on this total freedom? There has to be some mutual understanding and giving on both sides.

Vas and Tubal Ligations

A brief discussion of vas and tubal ligation is included here to correct any misinformation you may have and for one other reason (see below).

The vas deferens is a tube leading from the testes to the urethra in the male, carrying the sperm from the testes to the urethra. It is a firm structure, somewhat less than one-quarter inch in diameter, which can be felt bilaterally in the scrotum and is lateral to the base of the penis. Ligation (cutting and tying) of the vas under local anesthesia should be considered a permanent procedure. Reanastomosis (reuniting) of the vas can be done, requiring two or three days in the hospital, but there is evidence that the chronic obstruction in the portion of the conducting system at the level of the testis, not in the testis itself, sometimes affects the kind of sperm one gets after reanastomosis; that is, fertility cannot be guaranteed even with a reopened vas. Vas ligation does not affect the ejaculate;

it only keeps the sperm from entering the ejaculate. The 1 cm. scar is not apparent nor can the point of tying be felt except by an expert.

A note of caution for males: The first few ejaculates, postvasectomy, may contain active sperm. Contraception is necessary until the ejaculate is free of sperm.

A note of caution for females: If you find yourself with someone who says that he has had a vas ligation, you should assume that he is either 1) married, separated, or divorced; or 2) if none of the above, lying. Therefore, if you do not know him well enough to trust him, we suggest that you use your usual contraceptive until the relationshop matures to the point of trust.

The same approach should be used with the male who says, "don't worry, my sperm count is so low that I was told that I couldn't get anyone pregnant." In this case, we suggest that you use a contraceptive until after you marry him and thereafter as necessary.

The vas ligation and the low sperm count are classic, though infrequent, "lines" with the casual encounter or one-night stand, whom you will never see again. They sound like wild stories, but we have heard them, and our 80-year-old mother-in-law, a physician in New Haven who has been seeing pregnant adolescents, late teens, and girls in their twenties for 50 years, has heard them many times.

Tubal ligation involves cutting, separating, and tying the Fallopian tubes which carry the egg, fertilized or not, from the ovary to the uterus. Fertilization occurs in the tube. Ligation can be done through the abdominal wall or, in most women, vaginally. It requires general or spinal anesthesia and three to four days in the hospital. Cauterization of tubes is a recent development which is technically quicker and done through a minimal incision in the abdomen; it still requires the same anesthesia, though the hospitalization may be only a single day or an overnight stay. Some gynecologists are proficient in ligating tubes via the vaginal route under local anesthesia.

In general, women who have had their tubes tied are either married, separated, or divorced.

Reuniting the tubes is a major surgical procedure and only successful in expert and experienced hands. Success is defined as the presence of open tubes. Tubal ligation has no effect on subsequent ova, if the tubes are reanastomosed, but open tubes do not guarantee pregnancy. Fertility potential changes from year to year, or may change whether tubes are open or closed.

Male and female tubal ligations are relatively simple procedures, more so in the male, and any urologist or gynecologist can do them. The difficulty arises with reanastomosis, and at present the number of urologists and gynecologists trained and experienced in this field is relatively small.

Rhythm

QUESTION: I am 19 and have very regular periods. My steady, who is a freshman in medical school, tells me that we can use rhythm. I do not know how it works because it wasn't explained very well. Is it reliable?

ANSWER: If you are talking about 100 percent contraception, as we assume you are, it isn't. It isn't even 50 percent reliable. Nor will douching, which is not a method of contraception, improve these percentages. Sperm have been found in the cervical mucus 15 to 20 seconds after they have been deposited. There are good reasons for calling rhythm a form of Russian or even "Vatican" roulette, which is one chance out of six. A woman ovulates about 500 eggs during the 30-plus years of her reproductive life. If she has intercourse on the average of twice a week for these 30 years (about 3,000 times), an average of one out of every six encounters has reproductive potential!

Rhythm is a method of contraception based on avoiding the time of ovulation. Ovulation occurs once a month, or more accurately, it occurs once in each menstrual cycle, whatever the length. There is a period of one to three days at the time of ovulation during which the egg may be fertilized. A point of interest here: Mothers who are breast-feeding their babies do not usually menstruate, but they can and do ovulate at least once prior to their first menstrual period after delivery. This may occur while the mother is still nursing. Some girls have spotting (bleeding) at the time of ovulation, some have mild to severe cramping, but most have no signs or symptoms at all (see p. 26). A degree rise in the basal body temperature occurs with ovulation but that determination requires taking the temperature every morning before arising. (Increases in temperature may occur for other reasons, which may cause some confusion.)

The basic problem with using the rhythm method is that in the late teens and early twenties, girls cannot predict the beginning of their next menstrual cycle, or Day 1. The time of ovulation can only be determined retrospectively from this date, that is 14 days *before* the first day of the next menstrual period, not 12 to 14 days *after* the first day, as many people suppose.

The vital word is *before* menstruation. This means that in a 28-day cycle, ovulation is about Day 14; a 21-day cycle (which, if regular, is perfectly normal, though a nuisance) puts ovulation at about Day 7; a 34-day cycle puts ovulation at Day 20. Even a 40-day cycle is normal, if regular, and some girls are regularly irregular.

The obvious problem is that even normal menstrual cycles have a variation of two to five days, and in the young adult group menstrual cycles can be even wilder. It is a rare girl who can get through her teens and early twenties without skipping periods, having delayed periods for legitimate reasons not associated with pregnancy, or having some menstrual abnormality that makes predicting Day 1 of the next cycle absolutely unreliable. The saving grace here is that when periods become grossly irregular, the chance that they are anovulatory (no ovulation) is increased. But this is also uncertain.

So, from the egg's point of view, if you add the numbers correctly, there are at least six or seven days in each regular cycle that must be set aside as a possible fertilization period.

From the sperm's point of view, motile sperm have been demonstrated in the cervical mucus as late as five days after being deposited and in the Fallopian tube as long as seven days later. Some people question whether these old sperm are capable of fertilizing an egg, but every motile sperm must be regarded as suspect, for example, pregnancies after intercourse on Day 6 or 7 only.

In summary, assuming regular periods and their normal variations, you must add the fertilization period, at least seven days per cycle, to the possibility of sperm living five days, and then add a day or two for good measure. The result is two weeks of abstinence out of the so-called normal cycle, not including menstrual periods.

Regardless of your past history of regular periods, always remember that you can never predict accurately in your age group when your next period will occur; therefore you are almost never in a position to say that you have or have not ovulated.

Diaphragms

QUESTION: I have been thinking about getting a diaphragm because I don't like to appear as available as the girl who uses the pill, but I have read in the newspaper that "the pill is three times as effective as the IUD and many times more effective than the diaphragm." I have heard better statistics than that—almost 100 percent. Can you explain the difference?

ANSWER: We do not like those statistics either, but they are correct if we include the whole population of women in the reproductive age group. Research in the clinical aspects of contraception is particularly difficult to put into statistical form because of the uncontrollable variables—lack of detailed knowledge about usage; the surprising, brief loss of logical behavior which occurs with intense sexual stimulation; and with some, a subconscious desire to get pregnant. The latter may be evidenced by forgetting a few pills, haphazardly using the diaphragm, not checking before intercourse to make sure the IUD is still there, and so on.

Fifteen or twenty years ago it was taught that only a college graduate or a mechanical genius could use a diaphragm. Most of your mothers' gynecologists were in school at that time, and so were we. Effective use of the diaphragm has nothing to do with acquired learning; it is a matter of native intelligence and motivation. For the motivated girl, the diaphragm works well if she understands the basic principles involved and does not overuse it (see below).

Many feel that the diaphragm is an excellent method of contraception which is especially acceptable when intercourse is infrequent, as in the casual encounter, the one-night stand, the weekend affair. It is portable for only occasional exposure and avoids the daily pill. Save the pill for increased frequency and spacing children post-marriage. You have many contraceptive years ahead of you in which you will be using all of the methods available, plus some new ones not yet invented (see Pill).

Following is some basic information about the diaphragm which you should consider. Further details are really patient-doctor conversation and are essential for proper knowledge and use.

For those who do not know, the diaphragm is rubber, dome-shaped, and fits over the cervix, the vaginal portion of the uterus, and the anterior wall of the vagina. It is designed so that the spermicidal gels and cremes are contained over the cervix at all times. Some spermicidal agents may be used without a diaphragm, but its use insures the proper placement and maintenance of those agents. Using the diaphragm by itself is not a contraceptive technique. Neither partner will be aware of the presence of a well-fitted, properly-inserted diaphragm.

Diaphragms must be fitted by a physician; there are six or seven sizes. Refitting is necessary every two or three years prior to pregnancy and immediately after delivery. Some women who have relaxation of the pelvic musculature after one or more deliveries cannot be fitted. Prior to childbirth, almost all women can be fitted easily.

The diaphragm should be left in place for at least six hours after the last exposure. "Safe" encounters are limited to twice, with additional gel, for any one period of insertion, though some couples push their luck a little further. The diaphragm should be checked for a change in position if it is reused. There are always condoms for any greater frequency.

Diaphragms can be inserted one or two hours prior to intercourse or immediately before. In the old prepill days early in marriage, women inserted them routinely every night. Antipill women still do.

The argument that says "too messy" is not valid. For girls who do not like the difficult, slippery manipulation necessary, an introducer is available which allows insertion of the diaphragm easily and neatly, like a tampon.* Some physicians do not believe in introducers, saying that girls should get used to their vaginas. They fail to recognize that sexual activity often precedes any emotional comfort about self-manipulation and that in such situations "neat and easy" placement is essential. A quick washcloth will remove the excess gel or cream, and sometimes extra lubrication is a welcome thing.

The argument that says "too mechanical" can be applied to almost any type of contraception, male or female, depending on the individual's feeling about it. Some girls do not like to be reminded of contraception every day, the pill, especially if no male is available. They prefer to think about it only when it is needed and to forget it the rest of the time.

---

* At present, introducers are available only for the "flatspring," not for the arcflex type.

Diaphragm failures are related to nonusage, misusage, overusage. The last two "diaphragm pregnancies" that we heard about were: 1) a married woman with two small children who admitted that she had run out, and having had no time to get supplies had used what she could get from the bottom of the tube instead of suggesting a condom for that occasion, and 2) an 18-year-old girl who had had one spontaneous abortion, a miscarriage following intercourse without contraception. She had used the diaphragm effectively for eight months, but was in a hurry one time and knew that it was not in correctly. She is continuing to use the diaphragm after this last induced abortion.

We think that these examples illustrate the factors of emotion and haphazard use which make statistics on contraception difficult to interpret (see Douching).

In short, we can only talk about 100 percent effectiveness in relation to the pill because there is no ovulation. But even the pill is frequently misused.

The Pill

We are not antipill. It is great in the right circumstances, but before you are convinced that it is the only effective method, please consider the following:

1) There are really only two periods in a couple's sexual life when anxiety about pregnancy, in the form of preventing pregnancy or trying to get pregnant, doesn't lurk in the background of every sexual act. These are: a) between their first and second child, when both partners have proved that the woman can get pregnant and really do not care when the second one arrives, and b) after the woman is menopausal, at least two years without a menstrual period from the late thirties on.

2) There is no single contraceptive which is appropriate throughout anyone's contraceptive life (30-plus years). Circumstances change with the development of trust, with increasing or decreasing frequency of intercourse, with illness, with the number of pregnancies, and

so on. There is even a place for the use of spermicidal foams and gels and the IUD (see discussion of these methods). It is up to both partners to be aware of all methods and how to use them. Starting your contraceptive life with the pill has a tendency to spoil both of you emotionally for all other methods, and you may need them.

3) Premarital intercourse, at the casual infrequent level, is quite different from living with someone, with or without a license. In the latter situation, you do not always know if there will be intercourse when you go to bed, or are horizontal, anyplace; it may be 2 A.M., 6 A.M. or not at all. This is why the pill has so many advocates; neither partner has to get up.

At the dating level, or when meeting one or two times a week, you generally know that if you go to bed you will have intercourse, and you can easily take two minutes to put in a diaphragm. You may even do this before you go out, although they are portable. (Large bags are in style and will easily hold a cosmetic bag with equipment.)

We are uncomfortable with the idea of girls being sent to school on the pill when there is no male in sight and there may be no one for six to eight months. On the other hand, we are well aware that there are girls whom we wouldn't trust with a diaphragm or any other method. But, in general, these are the same girls that cannot be trusted to take the pill every day except in some crazy, careless fashion. Motivation is the key and lack of motivation leads to carelessness with any form of contraception.

Please consider the idea of saving the pill for the "living with" situations in your life and the first 10 to 12 years of marriage, when pills will be interspersed with pregnancies.

We're not enthusiastic about promoting abortions, but realistically, the present climate allows you to use something less than 100 percent for infrequent exposure. This leaves you weighing the *risk* of the pill against the *risk* of abortion. At present, most gynecologists we have spoken with are convinced that the risk with the pill is less. Condoms, diaphragms, and abstinence have been effective for a large number of responsible people in the last three generations.

Dr. Celso-Ramon Garcia, who was with Dr. John Rock and Dr. Gregory Pincus at the pill's inception and supervised the original Puerto Rican studies in the mid-1950s. gives two reasons for not making judgments about the effects of 20- to 30-year use of the pill and pregnancies on the individual female. 1) Any conjectures about effects would be only that, conjectures, and 2) It was demonstrated in the first 14 years of the "pill studies" that it is not in the nature of the human female to take pills for that length of time for this purpose. During that time only about eight of the original women in Puerto Rico and perhaps a similar number in California continued to take the pills. And they had to be cajoled, at intervals, to continue, not because of side effects but simply because they were tired of taking them.

He feels, and some studies have shown, that with the increasing ease of obtaining some type of permanent contraception in the form of male or female sterilization after the family has been completed, about one-fourth to one-third of all couples are looking toward this means of contraception.

It is his opinion, and that of many others, that the maximum use of the pill in this society will probably not exceed 12 to 14 years of intermittent use, that is, pill interspersed with pregnancies, and that at this level, for the patient with no contraindications, it is the optimal contraceptive method.

Briefly, the pill, in its various forms, acts as a contraceptive by preventing ovulation The menstrual periods that occur are induced or artificial; that is, the 20 to 21 day regimen was chosen to match the usual monthly cycle. Some women take the pill under supervision for longer periods, six, eight, ten weeks, or until a menstrual flow occurs spontaneously. They then stop the pill and resume it five or seven days later. This must be done under medical supervision, and it cannot be done with all pills. This allows for the juggling of periods in relation to special events like wedding days, and so on. However, do not play this game by yourself, or you might find yourself pregnant.

The secondary effects of the pill are decreased cramping with periods and usually decreased flow. The pill was used for these purposes long before it was used as a contraceptive.

The medical risks of the pill are almost daily items in newspapers and magazines, and only a fairly stable person will be able to read them and not be affected in some subliminal way. The statistics on clotting are generally regarded as accurate, but the risk is still much less than the medical risk of pregnancy, a poor argument in view of other available methods. The feeling about the lower dosage of estrogen being less risky is fairly well accepted but not completely, one reason being that different estrogens are used in various pills and their potency varies. Trust the gynecologist whom you see.

If you are on the pill, you should have a Pap test and a pelvic exam every year, or some say every six months. No connection has been established between cancer of the cervix and the pill, but the long-term effects of the pill are not yet known.

Pills are easy to obtain in most areas. There is no need to use inexpensive black market pills, or your friend's extra supply. You are only saving pennies with the black market variety which may be of questionable quality. Fifty cents a week will pay for pills, two condoms, or spermicidal agents to use with a diaphragm for the week.

CAUTION: IF YOU MISS THREE OR MORE PILLS IN A CYCLE, IN SEQUENCE, OR ON SEPARATE OCCASIONS, USE SOME OTHER FORM OF CONTRACEPTION FOR THE REMAINDER OF THE CYCLE, AND CONTINUE WITH THE REMAINING PILLS. DO THIS EVEN IF THE MISSED PILLS WERE TAKEN LATER.

ALWAYS RESUME PILL TAKING ONE WEEK AFTER STOPPING EVEN IF UTERINE BLEEDING PERSISTS OR IF NO BLEEDING HAS

OCCURRED. MOST "PILL PREGNANCIES" OCCUR BECAUSE GIRLS EITHER ARE WAITING FOR WITHDRAWAL BLEEDING OR DO NOT TAKE PILLS UNTIL BLEEDING HAS STOPPED.

The IUD

QUESTION: How does the intrauterine device (IUD) work? How effective is it? I have heard 98 percent, 80 percent, 60 percent. Which is correct?

ANSWER: We do not know how it works, but similar objects have been used since ancient times (see Norman E. Himes, *Medical History of Contraception,* Schocken Books, 1970). Its recent revival is due to the development of plastic material which causes very little tissue reaction. (The lining of the uterus does not overreact to its presence and no scarring occurs which might threaten subsequent fertility.)

The IUD does not prevent ovulation, nor does it interfere with menstrual periods, except initially in some patients. There are two theories of action: 1) Its presence stimulates tubal motility and speeds the egg through the tube, uterus, and out before fertilization or, at least, implantation occurs. 2) Its presence in the uterine cavity prevents implantation of the fertilized egg.

Insertion of the IUD is a two-minute office procedure which creates a moderate amount of uterine cramping, comparable to a mild menstrual period. Infection and perforation of the uterus do not seem to be factors except in the recently emptied uterus (post delivery or post abortion). A moderate amount of intermittent cramping and bleeding may occur for the first two or three months after insertion, or there may be few or no symptoms.

The difference in statistics which you quote is based primarily on the percentage retention of the IUD. It either stays in, is taken out, or falls out spontaneously.

About 70 percent of the entire female population in the reproductive age group will retain the IUD for a period of nine months or more. The IUD is about 98 percent effective in this group, that is, only two to three pregnancies per hundred users, per year, with the IUD in place.*

Only about 60 percent of the never-pregnant uteri will retain the IUD for this period (see Copper-T and Dalkon shield below). If it is retained, the chances are very good that it will be retained for a period of two years or more. At about two years, the IUD may become coated with calcium, and there will be symptoms of cramping, spotting, and increased flow. The device can be removed at this time and a new one inserted immediately or at a later date.

In the group that does not retain the IUD, it is usually removed during the first two or three months at the patient's request because of cramping and bleeding that is not well tolerated, or it is expelled spontaneously without the patient's knowledge. It is the latter which fouls up the pregnancy statistics.

The IUD is equipped with plastic or nylon strings that extend into the upper vagina. They do not interfere with intercourse, and they have two purposes: 1) to aid in removal, and 2) to enable the patient to check for the presence of the device. Some women check once a week, some once a month, and some always check before intercourse. The last seems the most logical approach, but a logical approach and actual practice seldom coincide in sexuality.

In almost all cases, pregnancies occurring during the first eight or nine months of IUD usage are due to improper insertion (see Dalkon shield below) or the patient's failure to check for its presence. If it is there it works, and it works from the first day of insertion at the 97 to 98 percent level, although some physicians suggest waiting one or two weeks before trusting it (see also use of the IUD with foam and as postrape therapy).

Dr. Celso-Ramon Garcia feels that the relatively high rate of expulsion and physician removal in patients who

---

* This is the only contraceptive which has a "built-in" failure rate even when used properly.

have never been pregnant is not entirely due to the irritability of the uterus, but results, in part, from their attitude toward the initial discomfort. He feels that previously pregnant patients are, to some degree, more highly motivated and emotionally capable of tolerating this discomfort and bother.

Dr. Luigi Mastroianni, Jr., has done much research on the mechanism of action of IUD's and uses them in individualized cases in his practice; but he says, and only somewhat jokingly, that they work best in a population without telephones. If the woman has a telephone it is much easier to come to the mutual conclusion with her doctor that the IUD should be removed than to tolerate it for a few weeks longer.

The crab-shaped Dalkon shield and the Copper-T are two newer forms of IUD especially suitable for never-pregnant uteri. The Dalkon shield is difficult to insert properly and equally difficult to remove. Pregnancies with the shield seem to be the result of improper or incomplete insertion. The instructions for insertion now include the warning that local anesthesia should be used with never-pregnant uteri. The Copper-T has an external coil of copper on the stem of the T which appears to exert some extra contraceptive magic. The T is small and easy to insert with fewer initial side effects and is less likely to fall out spontaneously, although some still do. They also have to be watched for a while.

In summary, if you are willing to tolerate some mild initial discomfort and to check the IUD prior to intercourse during the first eight to nine months and at least weekly thereafter, it is a very effective contraceptive, 97 to 98 percent.

Delivery at term is normal in those two or three pregnancies that can occur, and the presence of the IUD does not interfere.

There is no indication that the IUD causes abortion in the early months of pregnancy, if implantation in the uterus does occur. However, there are some recent indications that among those pregnancies which do occur with the IUD in place, there is a higher incidence of pregnancies in the tube than one sees in the same number of pregnancies which have been diagnosed early without an IUD in place.

Foams, Gels, Cremes, Suppositories

QUESTION: If contraceptive foams are not very reliable, why are they on the market?

ANSWER: Spermicidal agents like foam, gels, cremes, and suppositories kill sperm, but their common problem, when used without a diaphragm, is staying in the region of the cervix. Contraceptive failure with these agents is probably related to improper placement and insufficient quantity. We have heard additional complaints about leakage and taste problems, e.g., with oralgenital sexual activity. There are better methods of premarital contraception. But, like condoms, these agents are inexpensive and can be bought directly off the druggist's shelf.

There are two situations in which the use of foam, et al seems logical. 1) When you are really nervous and cannot relax unless you are 150 percent sure of contraception, use foam plus a condom or with the IUD. 2) When you want to get pregnant and have been on the pill, you cannot be absolutely sure that cyclic ovulation will occur immediately after stopping the pill. Some girls ovulate, some do not. If you are planning a pregnancy, go off the pill a few months early and use these easy, less effective contraceptives. You are then relatively safe and are allowing your ovaries to bounce back and start ovulating. That might happen immediately or three to six months later. A contraceptive failure at this time would not be the catastrophe that it might have been earlier. Remember, when you are trying to get pregnant it takes an average of three to five months, but when you do not want to be pregnant it may take only one unprotected exposure.

Research Methods

At present forget about the injectables and the implantation type of contraception. They are being used with some high-pregnancy risk patients but are far from acceptable to most individuals because of repeated breakthrough, bleeding, and disturbed periods. To a lesser extent the same is true of the minipill. A minipill has been approved for use but the pregnancy rate is higher than anyone who is reasonably motivated should risk (see Rape and Frequent Questions and Answers for current usage of the morning-after-pill and its side effects). The "Day 25" pill is still at research level.

Douching (doosh' ing)

QUESTION: Is routine douching necessary? If so, at what age should a girl start? How soon after intercourse should she douche to make sure of contraception?

ANSWER: Routine douching (washing out the vagina) is not necessary, but then underarm deodorants are not really necessary either.

A washcloth, and soap and water, used thoroughly, are sufficient until the time, if ever, that you become uncomfortable with a vaginal discharge. That time can be anytime. If the word masturbation concerns you, don't worry; daily use of soap, water, and washcloth in the genital area is not masturbation. Neither is douching.

Many women, maybe even most women, never douche unless required to for medical reasons. A large percentage of male and female gynecologists over the age of 45 are absolutely against it.

Americans are frequently teased about their preoccupation with cleanliness as contrasted with people in other areas of the world. With only a minimal amount of foreign travel you will discover that the sewage and water systems of some countries are not conducive to this preoccupation. However, in contrast to Americans, many cultures are preoccupied with genital cleanliness from an early age, for example, bidets, rectal washers in toilets, routine shaving of the female pubic hair, wiping out vaginal discharges with a handkerchief prior to intercourse, and so on.

Diaphragm users should douche before or sometime after removal of a diaphragm; the spermicidal gels leak out the next day (see Dyspareunia). In our opinion "pill" takers can keep the almost omnipresent yeast overgrowth associated with the pill under reasonable control by douching once a week or every five or six days. Many girls who are on a long-term, daily antibiotic for complexion problems could probably benefit from a weekly douching. (They also have a tendency to get vaginal yeast overgrowth.)

As noted earlier, douching is not a contraceptive technique. Sperm are in the cervical mucus as soon as 15 seconds and as late as 5 days after ejaculation. However, if there is unprotected intercourse on Day 6 or 7 of the menstrual cycle, douching may decrease the sperm population to zero by Day 11 or 12 (see Rhythm). In this situation, although thoroughly unreliable, douching might be considered a contraceptive technique. There is obviously no need to leap up and douche immediately; sometime in the next six to eight hours is probably soon enough, but still no guarantee.

The essential point to remember about douching is that it is not a major production; four minutes, after a little practice, is sufficient, and no bathtub is needed.

The use of the feminine deodorant sprays and foams that are so widely advertised does not seem to us a logical approach to feminine hygiene. The spray cannot possibly get where it is supposed to go. The genital area is not constructed like the underarm. They are not as effective, if they are effective at all, as daily soap and water. Some genital areas are sensitive or become sensitive to the chemicals in the spray, but this does not seem to be a widespread problem regardless of publicity. Since they are not necessary and are, for all intents and purposes, ineffective in reducing unpleasant genital odors, except perhaps those perceived at a distance, they serve no useful purpose, and provide a false sense of security for close contact.

Suppositories may be effective for vaginal "cleansing," but they only leave women with another type of vaginal discharge and do nothing for the external genital area.

The moist towelettes that come in foil packages are expensive, but they make much more sense than the two methods noted above.

It is our impression that the popularity of musk and similar scents among the "naturalists" is due to their strong resemblance to a clean genital odor, which is unique but in no way unpleasant.

NOTE: Male hygiene is equally important. As one 20-year-old female remarked after a mixed group discussion of feminine hygiene, "I think you should also discuss male hygiene, especially for uncircumcized males: they can get kind of 'strong' down there, too."

Timing of Ovulation

QUESTION: Is there a vaginal discharge which occurs within the last week or two of the cycle which indicates that the girl is no longer fertile until the next cycle and that intercourse is then safe?

ANSWER: No, but there is a vaginal discharge (cervical) which is associated with ovulation. This is really only of value to the gynecologist.

There is a constant secretion from the glands of the cervix which is conspicuously clear at the time of ovulation for a period of two to three days. If this is placed on a glass slide, it dries in a characteristic fernlike pattern.

The change in character of the secretion is usually not apparent to the girl, and therefore is of no value in determining ovulation, except to the gynecologist treating infertile couples and looking for the right time for insemination from either husband or donor.

A small percentage of girls have bloodstained discharge at the time of ovulation.

A slightly larger percentage have four to five hours of left- or right-sided pelvic pain of varying intensity associated with ovulation (mittelschmerz). It can even temporarily mimic appendicitis with a temperature elevation.

Most girls have an increased vaginal discharge one or two days prior to a menstrual period, but this is not usually very apparent unless they happen to be thinking about it.

As mentioned before, there is no really safe time when talking about 100 percent contraception. We are sure that many well-motivated couples are successfully using the last five or six days of a cycle as a "safe" period and that they may also be using the first five days of a menstrual cycle as a safe period, successfully. But in the late teenage and early twenties group, cycles can be so irregular that determining which five or six days are the last days is pretty risky. Even so-called normal cycles have a normal variation of two to five days.

The only other method available is the basal body temperature chart, and this is of more value for getting pregnant (intercourse at the time of the temperature rise) than for contracepting. Recording the temperature every day before arising makes a very pretty chart but is too much bother for most women unless they are just recording it for one or two months in order to get pregnant.

We are all waiting for that bright person to find the pill that can be added to the urine every day and will turn green, blue, or pink at the time of ovulation.

Pregnancy, Abortion, and Rape

Early Diagnosis of Pregnancy

A friend suggested that since so many student-hours, male and female, are lost because of anxiety about pregnancy, a discussion of the signs, symptoms, and the early diagnosis of pregnancy was in order, even though the question seldom arises in group or individual discussions.

Pregnancy may be diagnosed as early as ten days after the first missed period. At that time there is a small percentage of false negative tests but virtually no false positives. It is not really necessary to let anxiety about pregnancy rule your life much beyond this point.

For discussion purposes, we will assume that there has been unprotected exposure at some time during the previous cycle; this includes rhythm and withdrawal and partial penetration. The symptoms of pregnancy prior to and after your first missed period (see below) may be simply an exaggeration of the breast fullness and tenderness and the pelvic "awareness" that are normal premenstrual symptoms in many girls, or there may be no increase in these symptoms. There may or may not be mild, prebreakfast morning nausea. This is not usually the dizzy kind of nausea, nor is it associated with diarrhea. It is more like the nausea associated with hunger, and is often relieved by some sort of nonfat food, such as dry crackers or fruit drops. The nausea may also occur at other hunger periods, late morning, afternoon or evening, or not at all, and is very similar to the nausea some girls experience initially with the pill.

At the time of your expected period, you may have no cramping and no period, perhaps some spotting, or increased frequency of urination. There are rare instances when there is a relatively normal period, but these are uncommon, and you can only make judgments in the light of other signs or symptoms which you may have.

29

If you are sexually active, it is important that you "X" the calendar routinely at the onset of each period. (This is a good idea anyway.) If you have not been doing this, you will not know the normal variation of your own cycle which may be as great as five or seven days without your really being aware of it. This knowledge may decrease your period of concern by a few days.

Guilt or worry about that unprotected episode may delay a period. Worry about exams or papers or anything may delay a period. Girls in their teens and early twenties often have grossly irregular periods or skip periods entirely for no apparent reason.

But, if there has been unprotected exposure, do not wait for that second missed period. You might be six to eight weeks pregnant by then, which leaves little time to make any arrangements that you think might be necessary.

If you do not wish to be pregnant, here is one little-known fact which might be reassuring: About 10 percent of all recognized or diagnosed first pregnancies abort spontaneously in the first three months. About three-fourths of these occur in the first two months or by the time of the second missed period.

PROCEDURE: Bring a morning urine specimen in a clean, washed bottle to your gynecologist. He may do a slide test in the office in ten minutes or send it to the lab and you will know the answer in the afternoon. Most student health centers do pregnancy tests, both slide and lab, and do not report the results to anyone but you.

If the test is negative, you should request either an injection or pills to induce uterine bleeding. If there is no pregnancy, bleeding will often occur within ten days. Always get a repeat pregnancy test a week later, if the first one was negative and bleeding, with or without medication, has not occurred.

A pelvic examination at this early stage will seldom establish a diagnosis of pregnancy, but it will reveal whether or not you are more pregnant than you think you are. At 10 to 15 days, about all a gynecologist might find is a slightly enlarged, softened uterus and a cervix that might appear slightly bluish.

The menstrual and sexual history and the urine test are essential for diagnosis at this time. (Gynecologists usually count from the day of conception when they are talking about age of embryo.)

The introduction of this rapid, accurate, and inexpensive early pregnancy test has been a major breakthrough in the field, and there are several variations. Early diagnosis is absolutely essential for any abortion reform legislation to be effective. Because the method is available and inexpensive, a delay in diagnosis for financial reasons is immoral. A delay will also increase the duration of the pregnancy and the risk of abortion.

Criminal Abortion

QUESTION: Please discuss what precautions females should or can take after having had an abortion, criminal or induced, outside of a hospital?

ANSWER: Even in the present, liberated climate some misguided girls and their men are going to get involved in "criminal abortions" for financial reasons, so the question is pertinent. These complications may also be associated with legal abortions, but not usually for the same reasons.

Precautions should be directed at treating infection, and deciding when the bleeding has become excessive and if the abortion is complete. Do not assume that the abortion is complete just because someone tells you it is.

Any one of the above will require hospitalization. They usually occur together or, at the very least, in close sequence and may occur as late as two weeks after the procedure.

Infection is indicated by an elevated temperature, slight or marked, with chills, a foul-smelling vaginal discharge, or perhaps generalized pelvic cramping ranging from mild to severe, diffuse discomfort.

Excessive bleeding is one pad or more per hour after the procedure. Do not use tampons. Bleeding associated with cramping generally indicates an incomplete abortion that will require completion in the hospital.

Continued cramping, even with minimal bleeding, indicates that the abortion attempt was either ineffective or incomplete.

Do not be afraid to go to the hospital. You are not labeled a criminal in most states, and the law, where it exists, is often not enforced. You should be more afraid to stay home. Tell the doctor the circumstances and the type of procedure (curette, broomstraws, catheters, coat hangers, soapsuds, and so on). Knowing the method will help him determine the proper treatment and whether or not symptoms of a perforated uterus are present, such as internal bleeding and shock which may occur with some perforations.

Also, if you are RH negative, it is important that you be treated for the possibility of having been sensitized during the abortion attempt. There are increasing numbers of reports of RH sensitization related to abortion. This could affect the children of subsequent pregnancies.

Do not treat yourself with the odds and ends of antibiotics which you might have around the house or that someone is willing to bring you. Infections encountered with abortion run the gamut of bacteria and can even involve tetanus and gas gangrene. The latter two require intensive care.

The long-term complications of uterine infection are infertility and chronic pelvic disease, evidenced as recurrent pain, discomfort, and elevated temperatures. No matter how you feel about your fertility at the moment, the presence of infertility after marriage can be overwhelming, especially when you can trace it to the effects of an illegal abortion and your neglect of yourself.

The immediate complications of infection may be severe kidney and liver malfunction requiring intensive medical care.

Before you consider any of the nonprofessional, hotel-motel-apartment abortionists or any attempt at self-abortion with drugs, pills, instruments or witches' brew, please read the first two chapters of Dr. Richard H. Schwarz's book, *Septic Abortion,* in which all methods, their dangers, and lack of effectiveness are listed (see References). It is intended primarily for physicians treating septic abortions (infected), and can be found on the library shelf and in bookstores. You will be impressed with how well the embryo is protected. Having read this, we hope that you will not waste your time or life on any of the classic but ineffective methods, and that you will also realize that any of the drugs that might be taken orally or by needle have to be taken in such large dosages that not only the life of the embryo but the life of the mother is compromised. The fact that a method worked for a friend or a friend of a friend is probably fortuitous; about 15 percent of all first pregnancies abort spontaneously in the first three months.

Most motel abortionists only stir up the uterine cavity sufficiently to start bleeding and create a situation known medically as an "inevitable abortion," that is excessive bleeding and cramping with dilation of the cervix. The uterus does not stop bleeding until it is completely emptied. Usually the bleeding is so excessive that you cannot afford to wait the three or four days that it might take for the uterus to empty itself. The hospital is the only place to be. Some abortionists send you directly to the hospital after the procedure.

These abortions are usually incomplete because most illegal abortionists will not use anesthesia or sedation. There is an anesthesia risk as well as their own personal risk in having sleepy people staying around too long. Also, the procedure is really too uncomfortable for the patient to tolerate to completion (see Methods).

Consider the following example:

A missed August period, an illegal abortion in someone's apartment in late August, cramping and bleeding for ten days, no menstrual period by the middle of October (six weeks postabortion). When seen by her physician in late October the girl was 17 weeks pregnant. Diagnosis: failed criminal abortion.

In the student population an increase in pregnancies occurs about three times during the year: after summer vacation, after Christmas vacation, and after spring vacation, because girls either do not like to take their contraceptives home with them, or they become involved in unexpected "romances".

Complications of Abortion

QUESTION: If, during the first three months of pregnancy, a gynecologist in a hospital performs an abortion as a D and C, with an anesthetic, what is the risk of: 1) perforation of the uterus, and 2) infection leading to sterility?

ANSWER: The risk of either occurring is minimal. For all practical purposes, perforation of the uterus is potentially dangerous only when it goes unrecognized. This is why most physicians want you in the hospital for at least 18 hours after the procedure or with someone who will stay with you continuously during that time. Infection is dangerous only if it is not diagnosed and treated promptly. We cannot find any studies regarding fertility after therapeutic abortion except for a few figures out of some European countries that appear to show an increase in the incidence of premature deliveries (six to seven months) in subsequent pregnancies resulting from an "incompetent cervix" in those patients who have had previous abortions. The incompetent cervix simply means that the cervix dilates prematurely during the pregnancy instead of waiting nine months. The unproven implication here is that damage to the cervix occurred during the abortion. These countries have been doing relatively late abortions from below, vaginally, with mechanical dilatation. Repeat therapeutic abortions are being seen. There is a tremendous population for study building up now, and soon there should be an answer regarding fertility after therapeutic abortions, with and without complications. However, even without such studies, infertility specialists are beginning to see more patients with infertility problems directly related to previous abortions, legal and illegal, and to the increasing prevalence of gonorrhea, treated and untreated.

More immediate concerns are the risks with anesthesia, or postoperative phlebitis in the pelvis or legs.* There is also the problem of Rh sensitization, especially with late abortions, which might affect future children. Abortions are not benign procedures. We know of one death in Philadelphia that occurred after an abortion done under optimal conditions. The cause was apparently not related to any of the above complications and is still unknown. There have also been at least two emergency hysterectomies, removal of the uterus, done to stop the bleeding from perforated uteri.

Two factors must be considered when reading about the low rate of complications from walk-in clinic vs. hospital abortions: 1) There is little or no followup on out-of-state patients who use these facilities (almost 50 percent of the patients in some New York clinics), and 2) hospital abortions are usually later abortions and automatically carry a higher complication rate.

Therapeutic Abortion

QUESTION: How easy are hospital abortions to come by; that is, what is the estimated percentage of practitioners who would agree to do one given a woman who could pay and seemed seriously intent on not carrying the baby?

ANSWER: Let us preface any comment about the physician's role with the following: Any private physician has the prerogative of not treating a patient if he does not wish

---

*Phlebitis—inflamed veins with blood clots (thombi).

to do so. However, in the face of disease and if he has been consulted in his office, he is obligated to recommend another physician. Even with the change in the law, an unwanted pregnancy can only be classified as a disease at the psychiatric level. If that criterion is lacking, in print, any physician may refuse to do the abortion, and he is not compelled to refer you to one who will. In actual practice, most gynecologists will evaluate the circumstances and either take care of you or refer you to someone who will. Depending on his personal feelings and his hospital abortion policy, the referral physician may or may not require psychiatric consultation.

Everyone has heard "abortion on demand" for a long time. However, no one can *demand* that an individual doctor do an abortion, though they can ask legitimately for a change in departmental or hospital policy. For once, it would appear that the clinic patient in the public hospital is in a better position to demand than the private patient with a private doctor. Again, in actual practice, there is usually someone who will do an abortion if his hospital or departmental policy permits.

This negative attitude on the part of most physicians exists for reasons which may not be obvious to the individual patient. Simply put, abortions are unpleasant to do. Even doctors who have fought the hardest for abortion reform in their particular area or hospital, and know that they are doing the right thing for the individual patient, can and do get uncomfortable with the procedure, especially when the fetus is eight weeks or over in size. The doctor, not the patient, is the one who sees and removes the embryo or fetus and sees the body parts in the jar attached to the suction curette. If abortions are done after three-and-a-half or four months, usually with saline injections (see Methods), the nurse is often the one who removes the fetus and lays it on the table. It is not like taking out a gall bladder or an appendix. There are also nurses and anesthetists who are not as emotionally involved with the patient looking over the doctor's shoulder and counting how many he has done in the past week or month. Your best friend, or your doctor, may refer you to someone who has been doing therapeutic abortions in the hospital, and you may just arrive on the day when he has had enough and has said "to hell with the whole business," at least temporarily. Don't push him. There is a new phrase in gynecology literature, "abortion fatigue." This refers to the physician, not the patient.

QUESTION: Why are in-and-out clinics so much cheaper than hospitals?

ANSWER: Very simply: 1) Most good in-and-out clinics are located on the "doorstep" of a hospital and are officially or unofficially associated with a hospital where their complications are sent directly and quickly for further care. Thus the free-standing clinics do not have to pay for the blood bank, operating rooms, extra nurses, extra beds, or have any expertise in handling complications on a stand-by basis. They also have very little overhead. Hospitals may sit empty of complications but have to continue paying for these emergency facilities on a 24-hour basis. 2) Hospitals usually have had only the late pregnancies for abortion which require more time and personnel. 3) Public hospitals offer paying and nonpaying patients the same services, and patient costs reflect this subsidy when no city, state, or federal funds are available. 4) Even hospitals doing early abortion often use more than local anesthesia for suction currettage, because they follow suction with a D and C to insure complete removal of all the products of conception (see Methods).

Private gynecologists' fees vary, but do not be insulted if the clinic or doctor asks to be paid in advance. There has been enough experience to indicate that this is often necessary. Many hospital insurance plans now cover therapeutic as well as spontaneous abortions, even those plans associated with student health services.

May we suggest that if you are pregnant, you consider

talking to your parents? They may have the money and the contacts and may also be much more aware of the changing times than you think, once you get past the initial disclosure. Most physicians feel much more secure if a parent comes to them with a request, especially if an "under 21" is involved, regardless of any recent change in the law about medical care and minors.

Also, any abortion, spontaneous or induced, is a highly emotional experience. You will need all of the security, love, and understanding that you can find, and this is what families are for. We are well aware that some families do not function in this way, but do not try to handle the situation by yourself. Confide in someone who is close and reliable, not the man involved, even if he is paying for it; he may disappear, after the fact. The combination of maternal instinct and rapid hormonal changes associated with abortion requires that someone be around to help dissipate the emotion. This emotion may not surface until six or seven months later at the expected time of delivery when you start wondering, even if only for a few days, how it might have been. It is good to have someone to talk to.

There may be those who will disagree with this, but the Supreme Court decision on abortions will eliminate for some the additional and often intense emotions associated with doing something which is illegal.

The crass commercialism of some abortion clinics is very disturbing, but they are legal and nothing anyone can say will keep the desperate patient from using them. However, there is now enough evidence that some of these "lunch hour" abortions are incomplete. This is simply moving illegal, backroom abortions to the sterile, legal frontroom.

Early abortions are often referred to as being "as simple as tonsillectomies." But tonsillectomies are not simple or riskfree. Even when done under the best of circumstances, both procedures have a very high potential for postoperative emergency bleeding, and the mechanics of each require skill and experience.

Methods of Legal Abortion

QUESTION: What methods are used in the office or hospital abortion?

ANSWER: The method is determined by the age of the embryo or fetus (the duration of the pregnancy), but the guidelines vary with individual gynecologists or their hospital policy.

The procedure known as *menstrual suction* or *suctioning out the unknown* prior to any diagnosis of pregnancy should not be used routinely on a monthly basis. The risks of infection and subsequent sterility are high. To use it without skilled personnel even at ten days past the missed menstrual period is risky, since it may be incomplete and only cause further complications. It is also crampy and uncomfortable; any thing inserted into the uterine cavity creates mild to moderate cramping feelings.

In the first 20 to 25 days past the first missed period, a gynecologist might simply do what we call an *eight-quadrant uterine biopsy* in the office. Using a small instrument which requires no dilatation of the cervix he will take pieces of uterine lining from all eight quadrants. This is uncomfortable and often results in moderate bleeding and intermittent cramping for a few weeks. A D and C may or may not have to be done later for a "missed abortion," that is, the embryo has died or been removed, but it, or associated tissue, is still in the uterus. The uterus does not stop bleeding until everything is out (see the final paragraph in this section). Because of the increasing availability of legal abortions, it is difficult to determine whether this approach is as widespread as it was in the past. If there is no need for a D and C later, it is one of the least expensive methods, but its original purpose was to initiate bleeding and cramping so that a D and C could be done without question.

Up to three months, the time of the third missed period, a *D and C* or *suction curettage* is the usual method. Dilatation (D) of the cervix and curettage (C), or scraping of the uterus, and suction curettage are usually done in the hospital under general anesthesia. Anesthesia is used because dilatation of the cervix is extremely painful, but necessary to get a decent-sized curette into the uterus. Curetting the lining of the uterine cavity without anesthesia feels like severe menstrual cramping—it is not unusual to get cold, gray, and clammy when it is done—but it is less uncomfortable than dilatation.

Some doctors do D and C's under local anesthesia as an office procedure or in the hospital. The anesthetic is injected vaginally, on either side of the cervix, and only anesthetizes the dilatation procedure, not the uterine curettage. Oral or intramuscular medication will decrease but not eliminate the pain of curettage.

Suction curettage requires dilatation of the cervix to accommodate the suction tube. Some gynecologists feel that there is no technical advantage to suction over the D and C, except, perhaps, that the risk of perforation by inexperienced hands is lessened. Others feel that bleeding and risk of infection are reduced because there is no repeated reinsertion of a curette. Another advantage, some feel, is that the attending physician does not have to pull out the separate fetal parts of the later pregnancy with a curette; they just go through the suction tube and into the jar.

Between three and four months, the third and fourth missed periods, is a limbo land. Girls are often surprised when told to come back in two or three weeks for a *saline* (see below). The uterus is too large and thin-walled to curette safely and not large enough to inject saline safely. Injection of saline solution into some area other than the amnionic cavity may have dangerous and lethal consequences. Some hardy souls may do D and C's or, more often, suction curettages, but from three-and-a-half to four months on, most doctors prefer *salting out* or *hysterotomy.*

Salting out is injecting saline (salt) solution into the

fluid surrounding the fetus (amnionic cavity) through the abdominal wall or from below (vaginally). The fetus dies, the uterus starts contracting during the next 24 to 36 hours, and a dead fetus is delivered from below, usually in the hospital bed.

A hysterotomy is removing the fetus from above, via an abdominal and uterine incision. This corresponds to an early Caesarian section, and may have some of the same consequences in terms of the next pregnancy, that is, a need for a repeat "section" because of a weakened area in the uterine wall.

The former method is preferred by those who have some experience with it because 1) it avoids major abdominal surgery and a scar in the uterus which might be important in later childbearing, 2) at this late date it is more comfortable for the doctor to deliver a dead fetus than to deliver a moving one, which although it does not survive for very long outside of the uterus, still is moving, nonetheless, and 3) delivery of the fetus from below, with a minimal amount of mechanical cervical manipulation is always better for the uterus than any other method.

Packing is usually reserved for late pregnancies, when the cervix is softer and easier to manipulate. It involves inserting any one of a number of sterile items through the cervical canal and into the area between the amnionic sac (bag of fluid surrounding the fetus) and the uterine wall. This usually stimulates the onset of labor and the premature delivery of a living fetus. The risk of uterine infection with this method is greater than with the other methods described, and for this reason it is not used in the United States, except in special circumstances.

Rupture of the membranes refers to breaking the bag of fluid surrounding the fetus, from below, which, hopefully, will stimulate the onset of labor. It does not always do this. If it does not, other medications must be used, intramuscularly or intravenously, to stimulate labor. The risk of uterine infection is also increased.

The use of injectable substances (prostaglandins) to induce labor, with no mechanical intervention, is still being investigated and has many unpleasant side effects on muscles other than the uterine muscle.

Personally, if we were to have an abortion beyond the first 25 days, we would like to be lying right next to the blood bank. If it were done outside of a hospital before 25 days, we wouldn't leave town for three to four weeks, or go far away from a hospital. If the uterus starts to bleed after an incomplete abortion, it really bleeds, though this does not happen that frequently.

See Complications of Abortion.

See, PLEASE, Early Diagnosis of Pregnancy.

Rape

QUESTION: Is it necessary for all rape victims to go to the hospital even if there is no real physical harm?

ANSWER: Yes, and sooner rather than later. For legal reasons, a vaginal smear is taken to demonstrate the presence or absence of spermatozoa. In the case of attempted rape with ejaculation and no penetration, the sooner you get to the hospital the better the chances are of demonstrating sperm from the external area. Without the above, you have no legal case unless the doctor can testify that the physical evidence of trauma is sufficient to indicate an attempt. In this latter instance, there may be bruises and evidence of bleeding as a result of forcible entry or attempted entry. Bruises on other areas of the body should also be noted for legal reasons. This bleeding may occur even in obviously nonvirginal women and may look quite overwhelming for a time, but it may stop spontaneously or respond quickly to treatment (primarily pressure) and the area heals promptly without permanent physical evidence or damage.

More important, are the immediate concerns about pregnancy, venereal disease, and the psyche.

Pregnancy is always a possibility and usually can be prevented by giving large doses of hormones which stir up the uterine lining so that the fertilized ovum cannot implant. If you have religious qualms about doing anything to prevent implantation, you need not accept this treatment. On the other hand, if the hospital you are in has religious qualms about this kind of therapy, find a hospital or gynecologist the next day who will treat you. The treatment can be unpleasant, because of nausea which may be rather marked for a few days. For this reason the "morning-after-pill" is not practical or acceptable yet, nor is it 100 percent effective (see p. 87).

Venereal disease, primarily gonorrhea and syphilis, is also always a good possibility and can be prevented with antibiotics. This treatment is based on the assumption that you have acquired the disease at the time of the attack. If you happen to be seen by someone who treats only gonorrhea, he will ask you to come back for a blood test for syphilis in about six or eight weeks. If so, go back. Do not assume that you did not get the disease, just because you have seen no evidence of it.

The treatment of the psyche will vary with the individual. Some may need only mild sedation to get them comfortably through the period of nausea from the hormones. Some may require a short time on tranquilizers; others, long-term medication and psychotherapy. Some may need treatment for shock and require brief hospitalization. The gynecology emergency services of most university hospitals offer the above as routine therapy of rape with your own options, as noted.

The last point, and the one that probably prompted the question stems from stories which describe the lack of empathy on the part of the police and the doctors in the emergency room. We like to think that the normal curve of behavior in this area is skewed toward empathy in any group that deals as routinely and intimately as they do with this problem. But there are those who like to play father and mother even before they hear the entire story and "scold" you for being alone on the streets at 10 or 11 P.M., for not locking your door, for letting strangers in, for not taking normal precautions, or for hitchhiking. A point to consider on their behalf is that they do have to separate true rape from enticement or a variation of the latter. There are those who cry "rape" falsely for reasons best known to themselves. This has a jading effect on the people who see these patients frequently.

If the thought of having to answer such questions bothers you or you feel that they are not apropos, be reassured by the knowledge that you are getting complete and proper medical treatment. Then in the cold, gray light of dawn, ask yourself the same questions. For example, was I really asking for trouble? Was I being naive and unrealistic about the possibility of rape?

Rape is a reality, especially in an essentially urban area where potential rapists know they can always find women. There is no need to live in fear; but just as many people, in a realistic, reflex fashion look for exit signs in theatres and hotels when they enter, so, too, can common sense in this area become reflex.

Part of this commonsense approach involves prospective thinking. Instead of thinking, "This won't ever happen to me," think, "If it does and I cannot get away, I am not going to struggle so much that he gets enraged and tries something worse." Even enlightened police are beginning to say this aloud. Sometimes rape is inevitable, regardless of precautions.

Venereal Disease and Gynecological Examination

Venereal Disease

QUESTION: How much VD is there on campus? Is it really of major concern?

ANSWER: In any sexually mobile population venereal disease is inevitable. On any campus, the incidence of people who think they have the disease is probably several thousand percent higher than the actual incidence. It is difficult to determine the actual incidence in any population, partly because of the reluctance of many students to go to their own health service and partly because of the absence of reporting in the general population. This reluctance is slowly disappearing, but many health services have reported only a slight increase in incidence in the college population relative to that in the general population.

One physician at a student health center says that he sees 12 to 15 men a week, 48 weeks a year, who think they have gonorrhea or syphilis. This is one of 12 doctors' experiences with a male population of about 10,000. Of these approximately 750 men, there were only three proven cases of gonorrhea in one recent year. In a similar group of sexually active females, there were only four cases of gonorrhea and one of secondary syphilis.

Traditionally, the incidence of VD has been related to the degree of promiscuity, meaning more than one partner, and both have had bad connotations because of this association. Now, promiscuity is defined by each individual according to his own set of values and really only connotes that degree of indiscriminate sexual activity that creates guilt in the individual concerned (see Promiscuity).

However, the presence of VD still implies active sexual involvement with more than one partner, whatever the sex. Toilet seats, drinking glasses, and contaminated sheets

45

and towels do not enter into this triangle, or quadrangle, hexagon, or polygon, at any point. Reread Reuben, if you find a conflict here, and you will see that he does not actually say that you can get VD from toilet seats, he just implies that you can.

Patients are often unwilling to accept this triangle concept. Females with VD cannot believe that their best and closest friend or husband has been wandering. Males with VD cannot admit that their best girl or wife might have been seeing someone else. If the disease is demonstrated, facts are facts.

Venereal disease is really a group of five diseases. Syphilis (lues) and gonorrhea are the most common in the United States. The other three exist here, in lower but increasing percentages. Their signs and symptoms in the genital area are conspicuous enough in both sexes, to indicate the need for a doctor, so we will not discuss them here.

What are the signs and symptoms of gonorrhea in the male that send him to the doctor? These are urethral irritation, a symptom, and urethral discharge, a sign. The majority of the 750 men were diagnosed as having a non-specific urethritis, an infection in the urethra with no specific organism at fault as determined by culture and examination of the discharge.

Generally, gonococcal urethritis in the male has a sudden onset: He feels fine at noon, but by 4 P.M. experiences a urethral burning and usually a profuse discharge. Non-specific urethritis (NSU) is usually described as having a gradual onset over a period of two or three days with increasing awareness of the urethra, an itching rather than a burning, and the appearance of a minimal to moderate amount of discharge. NSU may be related to previous upper respiratory illness and have no relation to sexual activity or masturbation, may appear spontaneously with no apparent reason, and is common in some military groups. We mention these symptoms, not because they are absolutely diagnostic, but to allay anxiety until the discharge is cultured by your physician. It is worth investigating, even if there has been no sexual contact.

Many males are disturbed by the VD warnings which say they can have gonorrhea *without symptoms* and transmit it, as is almost universally the case in women. There is very little we can say in the way of comfort except to read below about what women have to do. Most sexually active women have access to gonorrhea cultures rather routinely, for one gynecologic reason or another, and their males should find some reassurance in this, if they can trust her to tell them.

What about females and gonorrhea? They do have a problem. The signs and symptoms may be similar to those described above, but those very signs and symptoms, in all degrees of severity, are fairly common in females for any one of a number of reasons. In most cases there may be no symptoms at all.

The girl's best hope is that the man will tell her that he has the disease and is being treated. The two questions she then must ask are "Was a culture done?" and "Who is treating you?" We mention this because of a somewhat sick practice that is not unique to campus life, and only slightly more prevalent than VD itself. The story is usually one of a "one-nighter" or a broken, brief romance that ends with a telephone call from the male saying that he is being treated for VD, or in a somber tone, NSU. Neither may be true. (This is called getting even.) The implication is that he caught it from the girl and therefore will not see her again. The male-female roles may be reversed, of course, although this seems less frequent. The only recourse for the girl is to ask the questions above, to hope she gets some answers, and then to investigate. If there is any question, she should get a cervical and urethral culture. Many gynecologists do not wait for a positive culture but treat anyone who has been named as a contact at the same time they take the culture.

If the cultures are positive, the patient is asked to return for repeat cultures (posttreatment) and a blood test for syphilis six to eight weeks later. The two diseases frequently go together. She should return for this test even if she has seen no evidence of the latter disease.

Despite the recent change in social connotations, gonorrhea (GC) and syphilis are bad diseases medically. The burning and discharge will disappear in a few weeks even without treatment, although most males and some females will be acutely uncomfortable during this period. It is difficult to say how much untreated GC progresses into the following complications, but it is quite clear that most, if not all, untreated syphilis does become a chronic problem, in some way, at some time in one's life.

Untreated gonorrhea in the female may ascend into the uterus and tubes producing chronic, recurrent, pelvic infections with temperature elevations, pelvic discomfort, and sterility because of closed tubes. With the increasing prevalence of VD in the general population has come an increasing number of cases of sudden, acute gonococcal arthritis, a painful swelling, usually involving a number of joints. Since this arthritis is also seen occasionally with infectious mononucleosis, it does not necessarily indicate gonorrhea.

Untreated gonorrhea in the male may also ascend to create chronic infection in the various glands of the reproductive system and the very real possibility of sterility.

Syphilis is a blood-borne disease, entering through small breaks in the skin and if not treated it remains in the blood stream for years and can affect one or several organs of the body long after the initial inoculation (exposure or lesion). This is in contrast to GC which is usually local, that is, in continuity with the outside via genital, urinary, rectal, or oral passages.

The initial evidence, the primary lesion, of syphilis is fairly obvious in the male, appearing one to three weeks after exposure, primarily on the mucous membranes of the mouth or genital area or in small areas of skin breakage, usually genital. This represents the point of entry into the blood stream. The primary lesion of syphilis is usually a nonpainful, raised eroded area from 2 mm. to 20 mm. or more in size, which looks like it should hurt more than it does.

The same lesion is present in the same areas in the female, but it may also be present on the cervix and hidden from view. More important, six to eight weeks after exposure, the blood test (serology) becomes positive and she may never have seen the initial lesion come and go. It is at this time that the secondary lesions of syphilis become evident in the untreated patient.

There is no need to describe the secondary lesions or the tertiary signs and symptoms which may appear either within a few years or many years later. They mimic many common diseases, a point made in the seventeenth century. These signs and symptoms will bring you to the doctor anyway. In contrast to primary lesions, the skin lesions of secondary syphilis are seldom isolated but are present bilaterally, on both sides of the body. Do not look in the medical books or that sore throat, sniffles, or rash will turn into secondary syphilis before your very eyes. Trust your doctor and hope that he, too, has a "high index of suspicion" that the signs and symptoms may be venereal disease.

The importance of venereal disease statistics, whether the incidence is low or high, is best expressed in terms of the severity of the disease when untreated rather than in the actual number of cases uncovered.

The coexistence of venereal disease and pregnancy is equally devastating for child and mother. Because syphilis is a blood-borne disease, untreated, infected pregnant women may infect their unborn children via the placenta, causing congenital syphilis. This is evidenced permanently in many visible and hidden areas of the child's body and physiology, and is the reason for laws in most states requiring premarital blood tests and at least one blood test during the pregnancy. Some obstetricians do a test early and late in pregnancy on all their patients.

Untreated gonorrhea in the pregnant woman may infect the baby at the time of delivery by direct contact in the birth canal or vagina. The routine use of silver nitrate drops in all babies' eyes at the time of delivery is regulated by law in all 50 states. This prevents the severe effects of the gonococcus organism on the eye of the infant, namely blindness.

Treatment is a simple matter of antibiotics in the proper amounts and follow-up cultures and blood tests. Please follow through on your follow-ups.

Remember, most student health services do not publish your name, put you on a list, or notify your parents. The very least that you can do is to notify your contacts or ask your doctor to do this. You must never avoid treatment because of embarrassment or get less than adequate treatment from the friendly local druggist. Your doctor is at ease with the disease and the contemporary sociology of the disease, even if you are not.

Most important, infection with either organism, treated or not, DOES NOT CONFER IMMUNITY. THE DISEASE CAN RECUR AGAIN AND AGAIN. Contacts should be treated at the same time and observe a period of abstinence, or the "ping-pong" effect will occur—the disease will go back and forth between two individuals. We have seen this happen.

The Hymen

QUESTION: My steady says that I couldn't have been a virgin, but I was. Do tampons break the hymen? I have always used them.

ANSWER: No, but they may and probably do contribute to dilating the opening in the hymen. This is a membrane which surrounds only the opening to the vagina, the introitus (see Figure 1, p. 102). Obviously, if you have been menstruating, there is an opening in it. Only rarely is it imperforate (without an opening) and then there is no overt menstruation. When you begin using tampons you usually start with the smaller size, and as your period gets heavier progress to the larger size, but even the largest tampon is only about one-third the size of an erect penis. This means that even this small amount of manipulation has caused some dilatation of the opening that is present. Even the hymen in a newborn girl may admit a fingertip. Also, there are many variations in the size and shape of the hymeneal opening, and some dilate more easily than others (see Figure 2, p. 102). The hymen does not break; the opening stretches and the edges of the opening which are membranous, may or may not tear slightly, with or without bleeding.

We do not mean to imply that only tampon users have dilated hymeneal rings, or that all tampon users appear to be nonvirginal. There must be other factors beyond individual variations in anatomy, such as exercise or manual dilatation during heavy petting, which have some effect also, but we have seen no studies on the effects of horseback riding.

Bleeding may occur with initial penetration and it is sometimes more than spotting. This bleeding comes from the thin torn edge. The bleeding may look profuse, but do not worry, nothing is really ruined and the bleeding usually stops by itself. Emergency rooms in hospitals see couples and usually give reassurance, or maybe a pressure pad, which the girl can apply herself (see bleeding with rape).

"Ease of penetration" is not the criterion for previous loss of virginity. Difficulty in penetration may be due to a tight, virginal hymeneal ring but it may also be due to insufficient time spent in the usual stimulation prior to intercourse, that is, time for relaxation and normal vaginal lubrication. This time varies with each individual: it may be 10 minutes, which is a little unfair, or it may be 30 to 40 minutes. In regard to time, you should both be thinking about the other person and adapting, as best you can, to his or her physical and emotional needs and capabilities.

If your subconscious thinks virginity is important, and you are feeling a little guilty or uncomfortable about your activities, and cannot really call yourself a virgin in the physical sense, try this epigram, it might help: Virginity is a state of mind. Or check the meaning of *chaste*.

Gynecological Exam: Indications and Procedures

QUESTION: At what age should a girl see a gynecologist for a check-up if she has never been to anyone before? How often should she see one after that?

ANSWER: Assuming that you have been having reasonably regular periods, and are between the ages of 17 and 25, the following are indications for a gyn exam:

1) Inability to insert a tampon, or the "lost" tampon (see p. 56)
2) Severe menstrual cramping (everyone has a different definition of severe)
3) Severe or chronic pelvic pain
4) Spotting between periods
5) An uncomfortable premenstrual syndrome (bloatting, weight gain, breast tenderness, constipation)
6) Itching vaginal discharge
7) The need for contraception or contraceptive advice
8) Painful intercourse (dyspareunia)
9) Premarital examination even if there has been previous sexual experience
10) Exposure during embryonic life to medication given to maintain the pregnancy (see MA pill and diethylstilbesterol (pp. 86–87).
11) Missed periods or irregular periods are a whole area in themselves. If you are in the age group we are considering you can miss periods for any number of reasons or for no apparent reason.

If there has been sexual exposure without contraception or with questionable contraception,
even in the form of missed pills, you should bring
in a urine specimen 10 to 15 days after the first
missed period (see Diagnosis of Pregnancy). If
there has been no sexual exposure, you can easily
wait until the third or fourth missed period, especially in the begining of the freshman year,
before being examined, as long as no other
pelvic symptoms are present. In general, endo-
crinological evaluations should be left to your
"home" gynecologist; occasionally need arises in
relation to the sudden onset of grossly irregular
periods and in that case, if necessary, they may
be done in your student health center.

Frequency of routine gyn exams varies with the gynecologist you see and you should follow his advice after the
initial exam.

We are assuming that if you have never had a period
before the age of 17 or if periods have always been grossly
irregular, 20 days to 45 or 60 days, you have already been
examined by a gynecologist and been reassured or diagnosed and treated.

If nothing else, please keep a record of your periods.
You may need it sometime.

Procedures

Avoiding a *pelvic examination* is understandable,
especially avoidance of the first pelvic, even among girls
and women who are sexually active. It is difficult to understand that a gynecologist can examine the pelvis without
getting emotionally involved. It is also difficult to understand that you can have your pelvis examined without
having some unpredictable sexual feelings aroused. And
when the doctor says "Everything is all right," you often
do not know *what* is all right, even though it is a relief to
know this.

Sensitivity about these and other feelings of the patient

is not restricted to doctors of either sex. They either have it or they don't. The doctor who does a slow and easy pelvic, allowing for tenseness to subside, may not be the one who will explain everything he or she is doing or may be the doctor who treats you like an ignorant child. You need not have allegiance to any doctor after one visit. If unhappy, find another.

The infamous pelvic exam involves examination of the external genital area and slow insertion of a speculum, a duckbill-shaped instrument with no sharp edges, which opens and expands the vagina but only slightly expands the opening to the vagina. This allows the doctor to examine the vaginal walls, the cervix, and any discharges which might be present. The speculum is removed, and the doctor inserts one or two gloved fingers into the vagina and places the other hand on the lower abdomen. In this way one can feel the size and position of the uterus between the two hands. The area on each side of the uterus is felt to determine the normality or abnormality of each ovary and tube. Palpating an ovary can give the patient the same sensation in the pit of the stomach that males get when their testes are squeezed gently, but the discomfort is seldom sharp, just a new, surprising feeling. Examination of the pelvic structures through the anterior rectal wall is often necessary; the pelvis is very crowded and the ovaries, tubes and uterus, and some of the suspensory ligaments can often be felt better by rectal exam. The rectum is usually empty of feces, if this is something which has been bothering you. A rectal examination is usually done if the patient is obese, or if she has a tight, firm, virginal hymen, or if more information is needed to confirm a positive finding. Many gynecologists do them routinely, especially in older women.

No one is terribly comfortable emotionally on the examining table or with the position that is required; this includes women having their 30th pelvic as well as those having their first. But nothing better has been invented. The drapes, the white coat and the fluorescent light serve a very useful function because they remove any possible sexual atmosphere for both doctor and patient. The shirt-sleeved doctor with a paper towel for a drape and no gloves leaves much to be desired. And since patients have 98 percent more fantasies than experienced physicians, the nurse "chaperone" is essential to the doctor, often more so, than to the patient. The annual checkup should also include blood pressure, Pap test (see below), and breast exam. Contraceptive visits should include a blood pressure and Pap test and a gonorrhea culture, though for financial reasons many clinics are not equipped to do this. And many patients are not willing to pay even minimal fees for Pap tests and cultures, so they go elsewhere and go without.

Pap Test*

QUESTION: How old should you be before you start getting Pap tests?

ANSWER: Regardless of age, if you are on the pill, you should get a Pap test prior to taking the pill and at least every year thereafter. In private offices Pap tests cost from ten dollars up but are often included in the visit fee.

The Pap test consists of gentle and quick rubbing of the cervix with a wooden tongue blade or a long cotton swab and putting the adherent superficial cells on a glass slide where they are read as normal or abnormal by expert technicians. The presence of abnormal cells indicates the need for further examination to determine whether or not you have a carcinoma (cancer) of the cervix. There is no clear indication that the pill, in its various forms, causes cancer of the cervix, but at present the pill experience has been short relative to total lifespan. A few gynecologists are at ease with continuing the pill after demonstrating and removing a local carcinoma of the cervix, if having children is still important. Many are not, for no proven good reason, they admit, other than being conservative with an optional medication.

---

*Named for Dr. George Papanicolaou

If you are not on the pill, a Pap test is not necessary until age 24 or 25, some say 30. You should probably start getting annual Pap tests at the time of marriage or at *any* time when you start being sexually active. If you are having spotting between periods or after intercourse, you should be seen at any age, although the former is probably the bleeding occasionally seen at the time of ovulation or from a small polyp, usually a noncancerous growth, on the cervix.

NOTE: One of the most common causes of spotting after a menstrual period in this age group is the forgotten tampon. This spotting is often accompanied by a foul-smelling vaginal discharge after two or three days.

Orgasm, Sexual "Inadequacies," and Promiscuity

Orgasm

We have a gynecologist friend at another university who sees many young adults professionally and is distressed by their preoccupation with orgasm, primarily its absence or lack of frequency. He believes that the phrase "the tyranny of the orgasm," used by Mary McCarthy in 1947, and perhaps before that, describes accurately the state of mind of many young adults, male and female, who are in their early phase of exploring sexuality.

There are some who would be content with putting a label on the "syndrome" and letting young adults muddle through. We could cite numerous cases and specific questions and answers, but we thought that it might be more appropriate simply to express a few of our ideas on the subject which might be helpful when and if the occasion arises in your life.

First, as discussed elsewhere, overt sexuality, a euphemism for intercourse, is basically reflex behavior. But the young are only gradually beginning to realize that a great part of overt sexuality is learned over a period of time with one individual, and may be relearned or added to with others, depending on the individual's sexual activities. Or, more conventionally, within marriage it is learned and added to over a relatively long period of time. We are not talking about techniques primarily, but about discovering the needs of one's physical and emotional self and discovering that self in relation to the physical and emotional needs of others, even making compromises at times. The need for compromises seems to be the most difficult thing for the inexperienced to accept and creates the most conflicts in the relationships with which we have had any professional contact.

Second, we feel that some people regard the heavy petting, with or without orgasm, of their early or initial experiences as juvenile, although they did not regard it so at the time, and quite separate from the "adult" form of sexual expression. But seduction or heavy petting is a very real and necessary part of the physical aspects of sexuality for most women before or after marriage and to a lesser degree even for men. This is more true for the inexperienced, unmarried couples where a certain amount of guilt, fear, and embarrassment may play a large role in preventing relaxation and a decrease in tension.

Seduction takes time and this often makes things difficult for the male and may lead him to think that he has a problem with premature ejaculation. The tense or anxious female in this situation thinks that she will never have an orgasm or, worse, apparently cannot experience one. Generally, this is really only a matter of learning not only one's own needs, but those of the other person, and of being able to communicate these, verbally or nonverbally, with patience and understanding.

Third, there are physical differences in the external and internal anatomy of each combination of two people, which even if very slight, require adaptation and learning (see p. 78).

Fourth, somewhat related to the above and of more interest to males than females, sexual techniques of seduction which work with one female may be completely abhorrent to another. This abhorrence may stem from as slight a difference as the use of fingers for stimulation vs. use of the whole hand, but it will prevent relaxation, pleasure, trust, and orgasm. Females who wish to succeed must be able to communicate this feeling gently, or they will continue to fail.

Fifth, the old idea that clitoral orgasm is different from vaginal orgasm and that attaining the latter is somehow the definition of growing up, has been discarded by investigators and enlightened, experienced men and women. But there are still girls who do not know this and who, having experienced orgasm with heavy petting (clitoral stimulation), expect something different and more with intercourse. They are correct; the total experience is more, but the orgasm itself, wherever a girl happens to localize it if she can, is essentially the same and recognizable. The girl who says she does not know if she has ever had an orgasm, has not had one, although she may have experienced the extremely intense, pleasurable feelings associated with vaginal and clitoral stimulation.

Males do not have this problem because erection, ejaculation, and orgasm are all part of the same stimulation, and may even be entirely emotional in origin and occur without physical contact.

Sixth, there is usually an optimal, if not maximal, amount of stimulation during any one time, especially for the female, beyond which orgasm will not occur without a rest (see p. 75). This does not mean that on those very active weekends and nights, females cannot enjoy additional intercourse. (Reuben calls these several levels of intense good feeling that may arise, "skimming.") But women should not get desperate if orgasm does not occur each time. They are neither frigid nor failures, and males should not feel inadequate in the same situation. There can be very real physical and emotional pleasure in giving as well as receiving, which is what human sexuality at its best is all about; both individuals have to know and understand this. Many temporary alliances do not have this emotional backing and therefore appear to fail in the sexual area. Also, too many grossly selfish demands by either individual may make the situation less than optimal.

Seventh, we have heard a rumor that there is no such thing as a female orgasm and several girls have told us that their sociology text says so, too. It does not. It does say ". . . of course, a number of females rarely or never experience climax . . . . Studies suggest that at least some women cannot tell with certainty whether or not orgasm has occurred . . . ." If we are talking about the entire population of women, this is probably true. There is a portion of the population, male and to a lesser degree female, that regards sexual activity as a relief of natural instincts involving about 10 minutes a day. The women in this group do not really have a chance to find out about orgasm, except accidentally or perhaps in the early months of marriage.

If a woman has someone who is willing to spend some time with her, who understands the sexuality of women and cares about her, sometime and someplace she is going to find out about orgasm and herself. Having discovered this, she will understand that orgasm is not absolutely essential 100 percent of the time to a good physical or emotional relationship ("skimming" will do, on some occasions) and she will be free from "the tyranny of the orgasm."

To paraphrase Reuben slightly, there is intercourse for babies, for love, and for fun. Obviously, they are not mutually exclusive, but the classification is a good one. The most important point is that intercourse for fun is performance-oriented (see Premature Ejaculation).

Couples who have been together for a long time do not label the occasional lack of female orgasm or the occasional premature ejaculation a disaster. Such couples understand each other, can laugh or cry together, have a sense of humor about themselves, together and separately, and understand that there are times for non-orgasmic, quick intercourse and times for slow, lengthy "production numbers." The male can say, "Sorry, honey, I couldn't get it up this time" knowing that he will not be maligned by a silence or a cutting (castrating) comment.

It would help if couples who are just getting acquainted at the overt sexual level could be just as understanding. But "understanding" almost always implies involvement and involvement is not always the name of the game.

Eighth, couples should not be embarrassed if they need the dark for good sex. Darkness is often equated with inexperience or old-fashioned embarrassment about seeing bodies and genitals or being seen. Actually it serves a very useful function: It removes all visual stimuli and limits stimuli to touch, odor, and sound. Touch is the primary basis of sexual stimuli especially for women, and darkness allows both the experienced and inexperienced to savor all of the touching without interference.

Male or female orgasm is a physical experience that is difficult to verbalize (see References). Women who have had natural childbirth (*supernatural* childbirth) have the same trouble describing this "fantastic experience"; perhaps because they are trying to describe the same thing. Natural childbirth, without complications, is an expansion of the orgasmic experience often including much of the auditory and visual imagery associated with orgasm under nondelivery conditions. This is quite logical because the same physiological mechanisms are operating, namely vaginal distention and total genital stimulation.

Demerol enhances this experience and decreases the discomfort. Even if nitrous oxide (gas) and some local anesthetic are added for the cervical dilatation, one may still have a successful natural childbirth as it is described by many women, though they seldom seem to have the courage to say "orgasmic."

Premature Ejaculation

QUESTION: Please elaborate on the causes, prevalence, and cures of premature ejaculation. Does masturbation have anything to do with it?

ANSWER: We hope that it helps you to know that you are in good company. Anything you may read on the subject will tell you that this concern is prevalent in the group of young, educated males who care about their women and are associated with equally "liberated" women who expect more from sex than penetration and withdrawal.

A desperate desire to perform well often creates

anxiety that impedes performance. This anxiety may affect the performance of a long-married male who sets out on an extramarital affair. It may also occur spontaneously, as a result of emotional or physical fatigue.

More important, the gradual realization that a large part of active sexuality is learned over a period of time with one partner and may be relearned with another, means that many couples may find themselves still learning eight to ten years postmarriage or later, despite the relatively large amount of verbal sexual communication between partners that is advocated and practiced today.

Masters and Johnson's book, *Human Sexual Inadequacies,* covers this subject (see References). Their "squeeze" technique requires a compatible female who will do the squeezing for her partner although it is not that simple. Most premature ejaculators in the young adult group are often with girls who are not at ease with the penis or male genitals. This means that 1) the male will have to do this himself, and 2) he should have a compatible female who doesn't question why he is moving away and apparently indulging in self-manipulation. Several men we have discussed this with say that for the infrequent occasions when the problem arises, they have used this technique themselves, successfully. If you really feel that you have had enough unsatisfactory experiences and that it is a problem, read the above-mentioned book.

Masters and Johnson also list and discuss the use of anesthetic ointments. Their opinion and that of two urologists is that they may work one time, and not the next, and that their use does not solve the initial problem because they treat only a symptom and not the cause which may be situational rather than physiological.

According to most experts in the field, masturbation has little to do with premature ejaculation. Masturbation is blamed for many things which have other causes or no apparent cause. Some people even blame the present "instant gratification" approach to living on the relatively recent acceptance of masturbation as being within the range of normal activity. However, Masters and Johnson indicate that a long history of heavy petting experiences without penetration or any need to control ejaculation is sometimes related to the problem of premature ejaculation. Perhaps if masturbation was treated as a learning experience (prolonging the time to ejaculation) rather than as a quick relief of sexual tension, the dysfunctional male might learn how and at what point he can temporarily stop the ejaculatory urge (see Condom).

Sexual counseling of couples who are dysfunctional together is often directed at decreasing the amount of *mutual* genital stimulation or making it intermittent prior to intercourse, or simply omitting intercourse as an endpoint of sexual stimulation for a few weeks and slowly discovering all of the other pleasurable means of sexual stimulation.

Premature ejaculation in the relatively inexperienced male is primarily due to performance anxiety in a culture that is increasingly geared to ideas of mutual sexuality. You should find someone who understands this and therefore understands you: being understood is at least half of the cure. Premature ejaculators should not assume that every attempted act of intercourse needs to be a failure for the female as well. If they do, they will quickly create a female who really does not care about them because she will see a male who appears not to care about her. Many of the nonvaginal variations of mutual masturbation are very satisfactory substitutes, if mutually acceptable.

Masturbation

QUESTION: I have masturbated two to three times a month for about the past three years, while in high school. I have dated a lot but never gone all the way with anyone. Now I'm sort of afraid that maybe I've spoiled myself for any more involved relationships I might have in the future. Does this happen? (19-year-old girl)

ANSWER: Many good people have written on this and related subjects (see References). The general consensus seems to be that there is no evidence that a pattern of male or female masturbation prior to or during a premarital experience or marriage "spoils" you or prevents you from enjoying or participating at a good level in two-people, heterosexual relationships. Of course, this assumes that all other areas of your life are within reasonably normal limits.

They do say that, initially, there may be some disappointment with the coital experience at the physical level, because the intensity and speed of the masturbatory experience are lacking. This may be felt by either partner in this situation. You shouldn't expect the experience to be the same, nor we suspect, would you necessarily want it to be the same. Human sexuality, at its best, is giving and sharing and often "just being." We would hope that there are other factors in your relationship which will more than compensate, emotionally and physically, for the possibility of an initial disappointment in the intensity of the physical aspects. But, if there is a little communication between the two of you, this disappointment need not continue for very long.

If you have done any reading at all, you will have read that women can teach themselves to reach repeated orgasmic levels and that men are hampered in this by a "refractory period" of varying lengths after ejaculation. If your own reactions during intercourse do not make sense to you in light of this information, we repeat: Masturbation is not intercourse and should not be viewed in the same way, regardless of the fact that there seem to be so many factors which are common to both experiences.

Dyspareunia (Painful Intercourse)

This is of such general concern that a brief resume of some common causes is in order; there may even be two or three factors operating simultaneously.

There are a number of areas which can be uncomfortable during intercourse or in attempted intercourse, but the source of the discomfort is seldom of more than short-term duration, a week or two at the most.

The two most frequent causes in females are 1) an unaccustomed increase in the frequency of intercourse, and 2) vaginitis. Vaginitis, inflammation of the vagina, may arise spontaneously or from the trauma of increased frequency; every vagina seems to have its own threshold for what it considers "too much," although the threshold changes with variations in frequency, and it often adapts very well.

Girls only recently involved in intercourse are frequently surprised to find that something that is supposed to be so natural may give rise to mild pelvic aching and/or awareness of the vagina for 24 to 36 hours postintercourse. They suddenly become aware of an area of their body which they were never aware of before. With experience, this awareness gradually subsides into the subconscious; the feelings are normal but often require reassurance. Males are frequently surprised to find that they often experience the same sudden awareness of the pelvic area, an aching or even mild, itching penile irritation.

Vaginitis may result from a combination of trauma and the presence of yeast organisms. Yeast vaginitis, with varying intensity of symptoms, such as itching, burning, discharge, is often associated with use of the pill, sensitivity to spermicidal agents, occasional sensitivity to the lubricant used on the condom, and the use of antibiotics for infections or long-term therapy for complexion problems. The physiology of the vagina may even change with excessive heavy petting and allow yeast organisms to overgrow. But 14-year-old or 40-year-old virgins can have problems with yeast vaginitis, as can diabetics and pregnant women. Uncircumcized male diabetics often have trouble with yeast overgrowth under the foreskin, and the inflammation can be very painful. This is one of the few reasons for late adult circumcision. Starvation diets, illness, and excessive carbohydrate intake may also be related to yeast vaginitis.

There are other types of vaginitis with similar symptoms, and most eventually require medical treatment, although sometimes the yeast variety goes away temporarily only to return postmenstruation. Occasionally girls have to go off the pill for two or three months if conscientious use of medication has not been successful; a change in spermicidal agent or the giving up of lubricated condoms may be helpful. Some girls will abstain from intercourse because of discomfort, some will not. Continuing intercourse during treatment frequently prolongs the treatment period which, in turn, prolongs the discomfort.

Males may acquire a sensitivity to spermicidal agents or to the lubricant on their condoms, if they use that type. This is usually evidenced as an uncomfortable rash on the glans or the shaft of the penis. For females, minimal attention to genital washing and douching will shorten the contact with these chemicals and perhaps avoid the sensitization.

Females may be uncomfortable with deep penetration during ovulation time (see mittelschmerz, p. 27), or there may be a temporary, fluid-filled cyst in one ovary which makes it tender with vigorous penetration. Acute or chronic tubal disease often causes discomfort during intercourse, especially during the late days of menstruation (see PID).

Vaginismus, an involuntary tightening of the muscles around the introitus which prevents penetration, is a normal reaction to the "quick approach"; seduction allows relaxation. Most gynecologists have learned to rest the speculum on, not in, the introitus for 45 seconds or so before attempting examination (see Gynecological Exam). However, 45 seconds is not enough, physiologically or psychologically, for most lovemaking.

Vaginismus is often associated with lack of lubrication, which is occasionally a side effect of five or six months of pill usage, especially the low estrogen pills.

Vaginismus which persists with adequate seduction is not within normal limits: its origin is primarily psychological, e.g., fear of recurrent discomfort, especially if there has been previous, prolonged discomfort for any reason, or guilt about intercourse, whether it is the first or the thirtieth time.

The tight hymeneal ring which cannot be dilated easily or has not been dilated previously, often only requires two or three weeks of slow dilatation, either manual or using the cardboard tube of a tampon with each insertion, for two or three menstrual cycles. *Forcible entry is never appropriate, even though you may have heard that there is always some pain and bleeding the first time.* In rare cases surgical incision is necessary or graduated dilators may be used if the opening is too firm or tight (see p. 51).

Promiscuity

QUESTION: How much promiscuity is there on campus?

ANSWER: What is your definition of promiscuity? Do you think that someone who leaves a poor relationship or one that has turned from good to bad is promiscuous, if they go on to someone else? The degree of physical sexuality in these relationships is not the only important factor, although things have changed as we are sure you are aware. We mentioned in the VD section that the word promiscuity has been re-defined in the past few years, at least connotatively. Like masturbation, everyone has his or her own definition of what constitutes too much activity.

We changed our thoughts about the word a few years ago, when we heard a high school sophomore say that in her school a girl had to have a steady to keep her reputation. If she dated around, she was automatically promiscuous with all of its bad connotations, that is, a person to be avoided. A physical relationship was implied in both situations, whether or not it really existed. The image of 15- and 16-year-olds getting caught in that semantic trap is intolerable.

We would like to declare the word obsolete, and substitute something like, "How much honesty is there in the relationships that exist?" We cannot really answer that question either, but honesty is certainly a better goal than trying to avoid the label of promiscuity, misapplied and misinterpreted as it is.

Our definition of honesty in this situation is knowledge of your own motivations for whatever you do. It means understanding why you prefer not to have intercourse until after marriage; why you think heavy petting is enough, adequate, or all right; why you think that close body contact from top to toe, in the vertical position is legitimate activity, for example, dancing in the 1940s and early 1950s, and is all wrong in the horizontal position; why you are living with someone over an extended period of time; or why you are "sleeping around."

Honesty also means that you can leave these situations when they cease to be of value to either of you; leave them having learned a little more about yourself and the other person (including his or her specialty whether it be Bach, philosophy, Victorian lit, or romance languages) and leave without the guilt associated with the label of promiscuity.

This ability to leave means that you can leave even when there is no one else in sight; this takes strength. Hopefully, you have gained a little more psychosexual security (ego) with the experience which will allow you to do this and do it without hurting the other person.

Honesty means sufficient knowledge of yourself so that you can handle those situations in which you "accidentally" find yourself with two different individuals for a short transition period, while "picking up" and "dropping", or when, as so often happens to upperclassmen in September, old friends and new friends may overlap and there is a sequence of "for old time's sake" and "for new time's sake" encounters.

These activities may create some anxiety and guilt. In moderate amounts, these are healthy human emotions which make you think and reconsider. (They can also delay a menstrual period.) They also mean that all of those ethical principles you have learned in the past and are still learning, are operating at some level.

But, if you cannot rationalize your behavior and think that you need professional help, admit it and get it. To seek help is to make an honest attempt to grow and mature. Giving yourself the false and relatively meaningless label of promiscuous accomplishes nothing and can be self-destructive.

To paraphrase an old saying: If you ignore history, in this case your own personal history, you are doomed to repeat it.

Frequent Questions and Answers

QUESTION: Is sexual contact the only way to get crabs (lice)? How do you avoid them or get rid of them? Do you have to see a doctor?

ANSWER: The best answer is probably close personal contact, which includes sexual contact. USPHS pub. #772, pt. VIII says that they may also be acquired by other means such as infested toilet seats and beds. Crab lice are the least active of the three types of human lice and their transfer is usually from person to person, skin to skin, though occasionally they may be transferred via clothing or as above.

They are classically found at the base of hairs in the pubic and perianal region but may also be present on the eyebrows and eyelashes and the hair of the chest and underarm, but seldom in great numbers.

All human lice are dependent on sucking the blood of the host for existence and without this daily nourishment they starve to death. This feeding creates a skin irritation and an itching. When you look, you may find small, brown-white, flattened things, about 1 mm., attached at the base of a single hair. Their eggs or nits are also 1 mm., are cemented firmly to the hairs, and may be felt, if not seen, as a bump or irregularity of the hair.

The individual case (not groups of prisoners, refugees, and so on) is treated with Kwell, a prescription item, which comes in a lotion, an ointment or a shampoo, or with A-200 Pyrinate, a nonprescription item used in the same way. All areas mentioned above should be treated, including similar areas on contacts. Shaving may aid the process but may not be essential. Shaving might give one a more secure feeling since the eggs leave with the hair. It is the best solution if your roommate or your dorm friends are ostracizing you. The areas should be retreated in two to three days regardless of what the labels on the bottles say, and it is a good idea to look every few days with a mirror for a week or two to make sure that the embryos in the eggs were really killed and there has been no hatching.

Hot water laundering and dry cleaning will disinfect clothing and bedding. If you find yourself someplace with out hot water or dry cleaning facilities, put the clothes away and do not use them for three or four weeks. The lice will starve to death.

We mention lack of laundry facilities because the primary source of crabs and other lice in the young adult population is the world traveler (Europe on three dollars a day, cheap hotels, and a variety of sleeping bags), and serv- ice organization worker (Peace Corps, American Friends Service, and so on) who haven't done a complete job with 10 percent DDT powder, or anyone who has been living in primitive situations. You should take two or three bot- tles of either preparation with you when doing this kind of traveling, not only for crabs but for the head louse as well which is equally prevalent (see below). Antilouse medi- cations are available in most areas, though some of them would not pass the food and drug laws in the United States.

If you are wandering about the world, it is important that you know about the other two types of human lice, not just because they are unpleasant and difficult to get rid of, but in many tropical and subtropical areas they are vectors of disease.

The *head louse* is found on the hairs on the back of the head and behind the ears, as are its eggs, though with heavy infestation they can be found all over the body. Treatment is the same as for crab lice and combing with a very fine tooth comb, a baby comb, helps remove the dead eggs and lice. A detergent shampoo like Selsun, for exam- ple, helps loosen the dead eggs but they can be a difficult problem. (We speak from personal, total family expe- rience.) The symptoms are an itching scalp and bites on the neck or head that look and feel like mosquito bites. Some doctors who are well acquainted with the problem advise washing the hair every day for four or five days in a row, not just the twice noted on the label. We agree. Those paper or linen towels on the headrests of public transportation are not simply amenities; they have a function. Head lice are more active than crab lice, and upholstery material is often a resting place between people.

The *body louse* is unique because it rests and lays its eggs on the fibers of clothing or bedding, particularly in the seams. It moves off only to feed and to transfer to someone else. When the same clothing is worn over periods of several weeks, it may become heavily infested. The body louse is readily controlled if clothing is worn intermittently, or by hot water laundry, dry cleaning, or storage for a month, and an intermittent wash for you, too, if you have the problem.

If the human is relatively nude, as in some tropical areas, body lice may infest beads and necklaces. If you receive these as a gift, put them aside for two or three weeks in some paper or nonfibrous material before wearing or packing them.

If you are using sleeping bags of questionable origin, bring your own blankets and lie on top of them. Apocryphal or not, several cases of lice at a nearby college after a 1969 spring sit-in were believed to have come from sleeping bags. Body lice and their eggs are killed by low temperatures as well as high.

This is a real and increasingly frequent problem which for most people is quite unpleasant and always accidental. It should not have the connotations that it has.

You may think that you will never need this information but pack it in your knapsack anyway.

No, we do not know why Kwell is a prescription item, but it is in most reputable pharmacies.

Yes, body and head lice are slightly larger than crabs, but where you find them determines the type and treatment, and the newly hatched lice come in several sizes.

Yes, thrift shop purchases should be laundered or dry-cleaned before using, regardless of the source; no one is immune. The potential problem comes from those who have been trying on the clothes before you.

QUESTION: If you are on the pill, can you get pregnant during those seven days that you are not taking the pill?

ANSWER: Not if you have been taking the previous 20 to 21 pills regularly. The pill inhibits ovulation. Seven days, after the previous 20, is insufficient time for the next egg in the ovary to ripen to the stage of ovulation. The 20 to 21 day regimen was devised solely to create a sense of normality—menstrual periods every 26 to 28 days. You may not think so, but most girls miss that menstrual period when it does not occur, either artificially induced or spontaneously (see Pill).

→ *QUESTION:* Is it possible to get pregnant the first time you have intercourse?

ANSWER: Yes, without qualification. The first time is no different from the fifth or fiftieth.

Beside the classic comment from some surprised, pregnant girls that, "it was only the first time," is another comment, "but I didn't do it very often."

QUESTION: Can the diaphragm be used effectively during the menstrual period?

ANSWER: The spermicidal jelly used with the diaphragm kills sperm during the menstrual period or any other time (see Rhythm). However, for some people the first two or three days of a menstrual period can be a good relaxed time to have intercourse without fear of pregnancy, except with 21 day menstrual cycles; and a diaphragm without spermicidal gels can be used, not as a contraceptive but as a "hygienic" device to contain the menstrual flow for that brief time (see next question).

QUESTION: Is it safe, in terms of conception and of health, to have intercourse during the menstrual period?

ANSWER: Yes, with the following qualification. If your cycles are every 26 days or less, then your latest ovulation day is Day 12 (26 minus 14). If there is intercourse after Day 5 of your period, you must consider the possibility of the presence of active sperm in the vagina (cervical mucus and reproductive tract) as much as five days later, through Day 11. If your cycles are every 21, 22, or even 23 days, you can calculate that the risk of pregnancy is very real (see Douching, Rhythm).

QUESTION: Is there anything unusual about girls experiencing coitus five or six times during one night?

ANSWER: No, though this frequency is probably near the upper limits of activity in the general population, even in your age group (19). Generally, this frequency is a self-limiting experience for both the female and the male primarily because of their physiology. Trauma, exhaustion, and lack of adequate lubrication take their toll, and the whole experience may even begin to lose its emotional appeal. Do not worry about it as long as you are physically and emotionally comfortable and it is with the same man.

QUESTION: About an hour or so after being with my girl friend (heavy petting but no ejaculations), I experience a severe pain in my testicles which lasts for an hour or so. Is this abnormal? Is there anything I can do to relieve the pain?

ANSWER: It is not unusual. There are old slang terms for this. The best solution is to allow yourself to ejaculate at the time. The next best, and only, solution is to lie down quietly and wait for it to go away. According to our consulting urologist, masturbation to the point of ejaculation at this later time is not effective in decreasing the discomfort, but several men have told us that this method is effective in relieving pain or discomfort. Try it. Also, we are told, taking a deep breath, holding it, and bearing down as if to have a bowel movement, is sometimes effective in relieving discomfort.

QUESTION: Do all girls have a clitoris? (Yes) Can you see it, or is it just a special sensitive place in the genital area?

ANSWER: You can feel the clitoris more easily than it can be recognized when you look for it, even with a mirror (see Figure 1). Literature describing the clitoris is full of words like shaft, hood, erectile tissue, and so on that lead you to believe there is more there than you can see. (The descriptive and romantic literature about the hymen as a structure can give rise to an even more distorted picture, especially as it applies to the contemporary, active, tampon-using girl 17 to 18 years of age or over.) In rare instances the clitoris is very conspicuous, so conspicuous that it is embarrassing to the individual, and usually causes her to seek the help of a gynecologist. In rare cases surgical help is required but more often simple reassurance is all that is needed.

The clitoris is a firm area about one-quarter inch in width, in the midline and anterior, at about the level of the underside of the pubic bone. You may feel just a firm nodule or a slightly elongated cylindrical structure. The end of the clitoris may be exquisitely sensitive to direct manipulation and even painful, a fact which males should be aware of. Pain will frequently destroy all of the pleasurable feelings of stimulation and bring a female quickly down to earth, making it necessary to start all over again, but very gently. This is somewhat comparable to the pain arising from rough handling of the glans of an erect penis in the preejaculatory state.

The position of the clitoris in relation to the vagina may be different in each individual, at least different enough to require some adaptation of technique. The same is true of the relation of the pubic bone in the male to the base of the penis. These slight variations mean that stimulation of the clitoris at the time of penetration might be by the male pubic bone or may require simultaneous manual stimulation.

This is the basis of the comment in the section on orgasm that there may be slight anatomical variations which require adaptation and learning with each combination of people (see p. 58).

QUESTION: I've heard that you cannot get pregnant if there is no female orgasm. Is that true?

ANSWER: No. Artificial insemination with husband or donor's sperm does not involve orgasm but often produces pregnancies. Another example: Pregnancy can occur as the result of rape and that is usually not an orgasmic situation.

QUESTION: Is it possible for a girl to pretend that she has had an orgasm and be convincing enough about it to fool a reasonably sophisticated guy?

ANSWER: Yes. If she is aware of her physical reactions during orgasm, she can usually reproduce them if she wishes. Some of the "skimming" levels of intense pleasure with intercourse can be expanded voluntarily with relative ease. But she should not try to do this with an experienced male without ever having experienced orgasm herself. Actresses have used the grunt, groan, and tortured look approach quite successfully (see Kinsey on female orgasm). Women should count their blessings; there are no absolute performance criteria, except those that she alone is aware of. Failure of performance in the male is quite obvious to both individuals and can be a devastating experience for him.

There are enough individual female variations of orgasm so that no male who is doing a fair amount of wandering can always be sure with any one individual. However, most males are concerned about their women, and if there is any question, they will ask. There are also males who judge their own success as lovers by the presence or absence of orgasm in the female. The answer to such a male's question is obviously up to the female; she knows him best.

For committed and well-acquainted couples, female orgasm on all occasions is not absolutely essential; therefore the need for the question does not usually arise unless there is a chronic problem.

Contrary to many writers, we can even imagine the occasional situation in which the nicest thing a women could do for a man would be to pretend that she has had an orgasm. This is not hypocrisy; it is situational ethics. But each woman must define her own "situation."

QUESTION: I do not wish to appear crude, but my fiance's brother just returned from Vietnam and he says those Vietnamese girls have muscles that American girls don't have. Is this true?

ANSWER: No, but some of them are apparently not afraid to use them.

Much of the activity of the pelvic musculature in intercourse is reflex in both males and females. If you become frightened with this "loss of control" during your early sexual experiences, some of this reflex activity can be suppressed to the point where it is difficult for it to return spontaneously when you become more relaxed about your own sexuality and you both wish that it would come back. This suppression of reflex muscular activity need not suppress orgasm, though it may decrease the intensity of the orgasmic experience.

You may increase your awareness of your own pelvic musculature in Yoga fashion, which is also Far Eastern, by exercising those muscles which you use to initiate and stop urination.

No, no one urinates during sexual activities. There is another reflex mechanism for that purpose which cannot be suppressed.

QUESTION: There is this great girl that I'd like to get better acquainted with, but she is only about five feet tall. I'm six foot three and 190 pounds and have always been with tall girls. I've seen this combination before, but I don't know anyone personally that I can ask. Could there be problems?

ANSWER: There are two questions here: 1) Will I crush her? and 2) What about the size of the penis and vagina? The latter is the usual concern implicit in this question. This is not a "position" book, but any position that is effective and emotionally comfortable is the one to use. There may be a trial-and-error stage, but don't get discouraged.

The size of the vagina and the size of the erect penis are essentially independent of body size and type. The vagina has a fairly uniform length of four to four and one-quarter inches, if there has been no term pregnancy. The erect penis also has a fairly uniform size of five to seven inches. This already looks like a disparity, but it isn't.

We would think that it would be very disconcerting and confusing for some young men and women to see the vagina pictured, as it usually is, as a long hollow tube and then to read that it is about four inches in length. The vagina is not a hollow tube. It is really only a potential space, like a collapsed balloon, with the anterior and posterior walls in contact. It is distensible in all three dimensions and will accommodate a tampon, a penis of reasonable dimensions, or a baby's head. This means that the walls are always in contact with any object in the vagina. Some visually handicapped girls, and some girls who have heavy or profuse menstrual periods use two tampons at once without any discomfort.

The length of the vagina also varies with position. For example, it is easier to check the cervix for the presence of the IUD when standing than when lying down, and the instruments used in gynecology for visualizing the cervix, with the patient lying down, are all about five inches long and should often be longer. This positional variation is usually greater in women who have had children.

The only temporary size problem there might be is at the introitus, the hymeneal ring. This is not as distensible as the vagina because of its surrounding musculature and the inherent membranous structure of the hymen (see Hymen).

Increased sexual activity or pregnancy increases the ease of distensibility, but even initially, there is seldom any gross discrepancy between the size of the penis and the size of the vagina.

We are aware that nonsatisfying disparities in size can exist, for men and women. If your sex is for love, you will find a way to adapt. If your sex is strictly fun-oriented and temporary, you should both find someone else.

QUESTION: I heard you tell a group once that if you

had to get married because of a pregnancy, you should wait until the third missed period. I didn't really understand why.

ANSWER: If the pregnancy is the only thing you have in common and the only reason for marriage, wait for that third missed period or at least the second. About 10 percent of all diagnosed, first pregnancies abort spontaneously by this time. Three-fourths of these abort by the time of the second missed period. A miscarriage after an imposed wedding would, at the very least, be disconcerting.

If the pregnancy continues, find birth announcements that omit birth weights. We have never understood why parents should be prouder of a nine pound baby than they are of a five pound full-term baby. It is simply not an essential piece of public information.

(The reason we use the word "diagnosed" when referring to these or any pregnancies is that there is a general feeling among gynecologists, based on some evidence, that the rate of spontaneous abortion is probably even higher if we include undiagnosed pregnancies. This is difficult to determine because of the relationship and similarity of early miscarriages to menstrual periods. It may be evidenced only as a slight change in the character or timing of the menstrual period or no apparent change. Don't feel smug because you have never been "caught." You may have been "caught" and never realized it, which we suppose is probably the best way.)

QUESTION: What is honeymoon cystitis?

ANSWER: Cystitis is a urinary bladder infection with symptoms of burning and frequency. "Honeymoon cystitis" is seen in women and is usually associated with frequency of intercourse. What constitutes "frequency" will vary with the individual.

Treatment is always a problem, because unlike other bladder infections, one can seldom demonstrate any bacteria and only rarely are white cells present to indicate infection. Most doctors treat this with antibiotics and perhaps something to alleviate the discomfort, because no one wants these bladder signs and symptoms to develop, untreated, into a chronic urinary problem.

The diagnosis of "traumatic urethritis," infection of the urethra due to trauma, is another way of saying it. If you have this tendency, and if it is recurrent, some physicians suggest urinating routinely at some time after intercourse. This does not mean leaping up immediately. The urethra in some females is situated right on the anterior edge of the introitus and is subjected to more trauma than those only a few millimeters more anterior towards the clitoris (see Figure 1).

QUESTION: I've just read about anal intercourse in Reuben. Is there really penetration? I don't see how.

ANSWER: Yes. As to *how,* the classic answer is *with difficulty.* The only woman we have discussed this with was a semi-private call girl in San Francisco in the late 1940s. Her comment was that it was very uncomfortable at the time and for three or four days afterward and well worth the extra money, though she never really got used to the idea. Masters and Johnson note that the circular muscle around the anus relaxes slowly after penetration so that anal intercourse is not as impossible as it might seem, but it does require lubricating jelly.

QUESTION: Is it unusual for a girl my age, 19, to be totally relaxed and responsive to a man? My steady and I read, sing, eat, in bed. . . .

ANSWER: No, remember the late teens are a marriageable age group. The ability to create and maintain male-female relationships is not determined by age, but is a purely individual thing as you will see if you look around you.

You may feel unique among your relatively small group of acquaintances who may have different goals and backgrounds, but you are no different from the larger group "out there" with whom you are not acquainted.

We only ask that you at some time consider how much

of this relationship is pure "nesting impulse" and how much is real. There is nothing wrong with indulging yourself in the nesting impulse; the security can be very comfortable, but recognize it for what it is. It may not necessarily fulfill the criteria for marriage, so do not confuse the two. Do not get yourself into the situation where you let a good portion of life and interesting people go by, during your late teens and early twenties, while you are tucked away in your nest, only emerging for classes. Someday you may look back on one or several of these relationships and call them learning experiences. Perhaps you know yourself and the situation well enough now to call it that, if it is.

QUESTION: What should you do if you swallow the sperm (ejaculate)?

ANSWER: Nothing. Don't worry, it is an essentially sterile, nontoxic, bland, body fluid. Some males are insulted if the female or male gets rid of it by means other than swallowing. But you know best in any given situation.

QUESTION: If douching is not a means of contraception, why does Reuben devote half a page to "coke douches"?

ANSWER: Probably for the same reason that he devotes another paragraph to emergency Saran Wrap condoms. If you reread those paragraphs carefully, you will note that he doesn't really say that either method works. But it does make interesting reading. We first read about it in *Time* magazine in the mid-1950s as an "old Southern custom." But it also appeared that most of an older theatre audience recognized the significance of a box of Saran Wrap in a musical about the "fifties."

QUESTION: What influence does marijuana have on sexual activity? I've heard that smoking pot can reduce sexual interest and also that it acts as an aphrodisiac. I'll appreciate any information that you have.

ANSWER: (from our marijuana consultant) The relationship between the use of marijuana and sexual interest and activity is complex. Many people high on marijuana tend to become reflective and turn inward, thereby decreasing their interest in others, including sexual interest. Many report that being high enhances sexual interest and enjoyment. One theory about this increase in gratification is that when individuals are high, time is perceived to go very slowly. As a result, they report experiences of prolonged orgasms. Marijuana does not appear to cause sexual stimulation but frequently decreases inhibitions.

NOTE: A moderate amount of alcohol helps to remove inhibitions, but with too much alcohol the male may have problems with impotence (no erection). For the female too much alcohol hardly matters if she is not interested in her own functioning, but it does make her forget about contracepting and makes taking chances seem like reasonable and rational behavior. Be prepared, if your alcohol or "grass" threshold is an unknown.

QUESTION: I worry about the diaphragm moving around. Is it safe to use more than once?

ANSWER: A well-fitted diaphragm doesn't have much room to move around. The pelvic contents are crowded. The "tenting" of the vagina described by Masters and Johnson is really only a few centimeters. However, if the hips are elevated during intercourse with either posterior or anterior penetration, the pelvic contents, including the cervix, do tend to move away and tent the vagina even more. The diaphragm should always be checked for position after intercourse, *without removing it,* and more spermicidal agent introduced into the vagina if additional intercourse is contemplated. The diaphragm should cover the cervix, which feels and looks like the glans of an erect penis. Many cooperative males seem willing to check it because they are as concerned about the risk of unwanted pregnancy as are their partners. Using it three times, with three applications of spermicidal agent, is excessively messy and unpleasant (see Douching).

QUESTION: Does the pill decrease desire? Many of my friends tell me that it does, but I've been on it for four months and it's great, so far.

ANSWER: Frequently there is a wide gap between one's intellectual approach to sex and the reality of one's background, and this may evidence itself in many strange ways. For many males and females, the risk of pregnancy, however small, adds an additional excitement and thrill to intercourse. When the pill is taken properly, this risk is gone and with it some of the excitement may also leave. There is then a clear commitment to the idea of sex for fun which may go against much of the subconscious morality that even the present young adult generation has grown up with. This may also be a factor in decreased interest after vasectomy and tubal ligation.

Similarly, if there has been even a moderate amount of premarital sexual activity, the marriage license may decrease desire. The excitement of doing something slightly illegal or immoral by local standards or one's own standards disappears when the activity is legalized.

QUESTION: Is it posible to get pregnant from the sperm on fingers inserted into the vagina after ejaculation?

ANSWER: If we are concerned about the possibility of pregnancy with preejaculatory secretions in the vagina (see Withdrawal), or sperm deposited at a tight, virginal, vaginal opening, and pregnancies in the latter case are not unknown, these sperm may also present a slight problem. A quick wiping off is sufficient, but some males are uncomfortable about wiping off their hands as if the ejaculate were somehow dirty. It isn't dirty, just risky.

QUESTION: Why are there no male prostitutes for females—or are there?

ANSWER: There are often references to the fact that this kind of male service exists, but not even the many books on prostitution devote more than a few sentences, if any, to the subject. Males have a performance problem which prohibits continuous or repetitive active participation. Studs exist, but performance is never predictable. (See Joe Buck, *Midnight Cowboy.*)

NOTE: Male homosexual prostitutes exist, but their services do not always require an erect penis on demand. Female homosexuals have a much easier time finding females who are compatible over a period of time, and do not normally need or desire the kind of impersonal services a female homosexual prostitute would offer.

QUESTION: Do you think the fact that almost 90 percent of all American males in the young age group are circumcised has anything to do with the amount of premature ejaculation there seems to be?

ANSWER: No. The erect, *un*circumcised penis with freely movable foreskin or prepuce acts exactly like the circumcized penis during intercourse. This means that the sensitive glans is entirely exposed to stimulation in both cases. Due to the variable amount of foreskin removed in circumcision, some males are not always certain whether or not they have been circumcised; but if they look around they will find that all penises look slightly different from one another (see Figures 3 and 4).

NOTE: Circumcision in females may mean a number of different procedures, depending on customs in different cultures. It is not exactly comparable to male circumcision; that is, it does not always involve removal of the foreskin (prepuce) over the clitoris. Female circumcision may mean removal of the labia majora, removal of labia minora only, or both labia; it may mean complete removal of the clitoris as is done in some primitive societies. The labial procedures are still done in some Middle Eastern cultures although the practice is disappearing. Why? There has always been a tremendous emphasis on genital cleanliness and "neatness" in Middle Eastern cultures and the flattened, shaved genital area is considered more attractive.

QUESTION: What can be done for males who are castrated?

ANSWER: If castration is due to trauma, such as war

injuries or accidents, and the testes are intact and are retrieved in time, they can be implanted under the skin, usually of the thigh, or in the remains of the scrotum. In such cases the hormonal effect is maintained, but the sperm pathway is lost, as in vasectomy.

Criminal castration is usually associated with sadistic mutilation immediately before or after the victim is killed by other means. Threats of castration without apparent murderous intent are usually just threats. Occasionally castration is the result of self-mutilation in a mentally disturbed patient. If available, these testes can be implanted as above.

The bleeding will appear profuse, but the blood loss, we are told, seldom exceeds a pint, and gradually slows with retraction of the small blood vessels along the spermatic cord.

Testes are sometimes removed in patients with advanced prostatic cancer that is hormone dependent.

Eunuchs are males who lose their testes prior to puberty and do not develop any of the secondary sexual characteristics of the adult male.

Occasionally the penis is involved in trauma, and depending on the extent of the injury may become nonfunctional as an erectile organ, but appearances can be maintained with plastic (restorative) surgery.

NOTE: Female castration or removal of both ovaries in their entirety is rarely necessary; it takes only a small amount of ovarian tissue to ovulate and work effectively in the hormonal feedback system. Oral replacement therapy is available. Women with advanced breast cancer that appears estrogen dependent may have both ovaries removed if their physical condition permits. Removal of one or both breasts in the female appears to have more of the emotional connotations of castration than does removal of the ovaries.

QUESTION: Is the morning-after-pill really dangerous?

ANSWER: The MA pill is not a single pill as yet, but several pills taken over four or five days after unprotected exposure to spermatozoa. In theory, these pills affect the lining of the uterus so that any fertilized ovum cannot implant, or they may also speed the transport of the fertilized ovum so that it reaches an unprepared uterus. The ovum either disintegrates or is expelled from the uterus. So, these pills are not a contraceptive; if they work as claimed, they are really an abortifacient if we consider a 16 to 32 cell fertilized ovum to be an embryo. Some people call the MA pill and IUD "interceptives". They have not been proven to be absolutely effective because their target is an "unknown," that is, an undiagnosed pregnancy. But, statistically, they work, although several studies have had only incomplete follow-ups on *all* of the patients treated.

The pills will never be used routinely by any single individual because of the varying degrees of nausea associated with their use. They are used routinely in most rape therapy and by many physicians faced with distraught women or couples who neglected to contracept or "broke" a condom.

There is no known danger to the patient in the dosage used. The implied danger is to female embryos born to women who have taken the pills during pregnancy. Two points are against this danger: 1) The woman who takes the pills is trying to rid herself of a possible but unknown pregnancy, and even if an undiagnosed pregnancy is already in the uterus, the chances are very good that she will choose to rid herself of that, after one missed period. 2) The dosage used is nowhere near the dosage used to maintain pregnancies in the past. Some female offspring of pregnancies in which the mother has been treated have been found to have vaginal and cervical lesions, some cancerous; these lesions became symptomatic or were found 16 or more years later. (All girls should ask their mothers or their mother's obstetrician, if possible, if the former took estrogens or hormones during pregnancy and be examined with this in mind, if diethylstilbesterol, DES, was taken.)

The delay in discovery of these lesions is probably related to delayed pelvic examinations and also to the fact that females are not often examined until symptoms appear. Symptoms and signs of female genital tract disease of any kind are vaginal discharge, pain, or irregular or excessive bleeding. The latter two should be investigated any time they occur.

QUESTION: Can those fellows with neck injuries who are paralysed ever have sex or children of their own?

ANSWER: A large majority of them can do both. Remember that much of the male erectile and ejaculatory function is reflex activity. An understanding wife or girl friend is essential, but if both partners understand that it is possible, are instructed, and slowly discover their own potential, satisfying sexual activity and children may result. Some of the lower spinal cord injuries still retain some sensation in the pelvic area. There are training movies for paralysed veterans on this subject, and the Veterans' Hospital in Long Beach, California, has experts in this area of rehabilitation as do a limited number of other hospitals.

There are females with spinal cord injuries, too, and they can give birth almost or completely free of discomfort. Sexuality is really in the head; much of the actual function is more or less reflex.

QUESTION: Is it all right for her, I mean healthy, to sleep with my girl without intercourse? We're engaged and living together but cannot get married for two years, and we cannot use contraception. (19-year-old male)

ANSWER: If lovemaking is frequent but without orgasmic release for either of you, both of you will be uncomfortable at times which will probably limit further physical contact for a while. Some of the variations of abstinence may be acceptable and appropriate forms of orgasmic release. Two years of daily close physical contact without intercourse is asking a great deal of yourself and your fiancee. You should be aware that there is a point of inevitability in sexual stimulation for males and for females, and be prepared with condoms, even if they are never used.

COMMENT: A comment from some male gynecology residents in their late twenties: "We are always surprised by the large number of unattractive girls we are seeing in our contraceptive clinic."

The sexual revolution has been a boon to both the unattractive female and the unattractive male. And as one very attractive girl said, "We all have times when we feel ugly and there is nothing better than sex to get your ego back, even if it isn't spectacular sex."

Coed dorms and expanded parietals allow male-female communication on a physically close, intellectual level that was never possible under the old rules. True personalities can emerge for better or worse. When casual touching, the primary basis of all physical sexuality, is allowed to run its natural course between two people who find they appreciate and enjoy each other's mind and how they think, physical sexuality may be the surprising result of what began as an intellectual relationship; physical appearance does not matter.

We have seen several intelligent but insecure, unattractive female virgins emerge over two or three years into secure, sexually active women. They begin to care about themselves, lose a few of those "freshman" pounds and wash their hair in some regular fashion. It is a good feeling for both males and females to be enjoyed not only for their good minds, but also because they can function as adult males and females.

This all seems a little more honest than the cashmere sweater and pearls dating practices of 20 or 30 years ago, although it also presents difficult problems but of a different dimension.

For Parents:
When Chastity Doesn't Make It*

Should unmarried girls be given contraceptives without their parents' consent? This is a question which comes up from time to time and worries those concerned with administering programs and deciding on public policy. At what age is a young girl considered a free agent, and what is the responsibility of society in such cases? Does it encourage promiscuity to make contraceptives available, and what is the proper role of a parent?

Faced with this question today I recall a conversation I had last year with a pretty young coed who was telling me of the fate of five of her friends. All had gotten pregnant during their two years at college; two girls married the boys (rather unhappily) and three had gotten abortions. My acquaintance decided that she had better go to the only doctor in town and get some pills. This she did, although she resented his reluctance and the lecture which accompanied his prescription. (He was a Catholic and very conservative, of course.)

The shocking thing in this story is that her state college health service would not give out contraceptives to unmarried students. Yet all parietal rules governing dormitories and student behavior had been abolished. Many students lived off campus and in many of those social circles every drinking party ended with couples pairing off for bed. (Obviously this school was in the boondocks since there was little pot and lots of liquor.)

Out there the sexual revolution mostly meant sexual promiscuity, not meaningful I-Thou relationships. My cherubic blonde informant told me that usually the girls just got drunk so that they didn't have to be fully respon-

---

* By Sidney Callahan. Reprinted, with her permission from *The National Catholic Reporter*, September 4, 1970.

sible for what followed. She, however, while not able to stand the crowd's scorn for her virginity, could not go to bed with just anybody. So she carefully decided which guy in her circle was going to be the first, (one always has a special feeling for the first).

Three girls were in on this particular coffeeklatsch, and since there was no disagreement over the picture of the campus I was being presented, I was concluding that indeed life had changed since I was their age. However, when I walked off alone with the third girl, who had remained relatively silent during the chilling description of local feminine options, she began to speak up. She just wanted me to know that it really wasn't all that bad here. She herself was a virgin and she and her fiancee thought it important to wait for marriage. Many of *her* friends felt the same way; *they talked about it all the time.*

Hearing her story, I had to laugh at myself. *Why do I always forget that nowadays it's the chaste who are ashamed and silent?* Having had the same experience now on so many campuses I'm prepared for this wide divergence of views *and the defensiveness of the virgins.* At the same time I enjoy the outspokenness of the unmarried girls living with men. Once on a plane I happened to sit between two young lovelies, and in the course of the conversation the one on my right leaned across me and shouted over the roar of the engines to the redhead in the window seat (whom she'd just met), "Are you living with your boyfriend?"

But the questioner mostly wanted to tell us the advantages of her arrangement. Neither she nor anyone else in these testimonials much mentions the advantages of pre-marital sexual experience, but they do extoll the virtues of adjusting to the way another person puts the cap on the toothpaste, or doesn't pick up his socks. Living intimately out of bed seems to be the major learning experience involved.

Anyway, in this particular plane conversation I could deduce from the blushing evasions of the girl on my left,

"Yep, here's another shamefaced abstainer." Such conversations over the country give me the picture of tremendous, unrelieved pressure to have sex before marriage. The majority of girls aren't enthusiastic but they can't stand against the tide. "We never hear the other side defended," they complain. After all, what chance do one's grandmother, Ann Landers and assorted Christians have stacked up against sexologists, *Cosmopolitan* and swinging clergymen of all faiths. Sociologists too, are simply recording in their "value-free" way the acceptability of permissiveness.

Therefore when all support for chastity has been removed from the society you must provide contraceptives as the corollary of free choice. When you give up chaperonage and allow young people after puberty to go about freely, then you must assume them also adult enough to have contraceptives available. Old enough to be a parent, then old enough to be able to prevent conception. Free to meet others in private, then free to privately procure contraceptives. When the chaperone has departed and permissiveness is in the air, then contraceptives had better be in hand. Otherwise, the present messy social situation will grow worse; more illegitimate births, more abortions, more pregnant brides.

I don't think parents, however, should give contraceptives to their children. Such a procedure implies parental permission, cooperation and control of a child's sex life. The whole point of providing a choice is to encourage grown-up responsible behavior and self-control of one's sexuality. Sex is a free personal matter in our culture and so the provision of contraceptives should be free and personal. There ought to be clinics and doctors accessible who will give out contraceptives to anyone who comes. (To keep these doctors from giving advice, however, is too neutral a stance.)

Parents for their part, should actively promote their own ideals, state their own expectations and standards *and* point out the imperative responsibilities resting on those who choose to be sexually permissive. If a child decides to act against his parents' ideals, or if he is afraid that he will succumb to temptation, then there should be a *third party* to go to in order to implement the next most responsible behavior.

It's that all-or-nothing-at-all morality that gets young people in trouble. Let's at least be true to our respectable tradition of casuistry,* when chastity doesn't make it. Making distinctions between best and next best is a price we pay for being a rational species.

_____

* casuistry: application of ethical principles to particular problems of conduct or morality.

References

GREER, G. *The Female Eunuch.* New York: McGraw Hill, 1971.

Females can read this book and discover that they can be gutsy and liberated, and still demonstrate some understanding of the male psyche. Males can read it and discover that females can be understanding, good in bed, and bright, without being "castrating."

JOHNSTON, JILL. *Lesbian Nation: The Feminist Solution.* New York: Simon and Schuster, 1973.

KINSEY, ALBERT C., ET AL. *Sexual Behavior in the Human Female.** Philadelphia: W. B. Saunders Company, 1953.

Still valid and readable in the areas of masturbation and homosexuality in the female as well as good reading on the psychological components of sexuality.

———. *Sexual Behavior in the Human Male.* Philadelphia: W. B. Saunders Company, 1948.

Still valid and readable in the areas of masturbation and homosexuality in the male as well as good reading on the psychological components of sexuality.

MCCAFFREY, JOSEPH A. *The Homosexual Dialectic.* Englewood Cliffs, N. J.: Prentice-Hall, Inc., 1972.

A collection of fifteen articles, some original for this publication, by a variety of writers—some research, some militant, some personal—including one long article on the "social and attitudinal dimensions" of female homosexuality with an extensive bibliography on this subject.

MAILER, N. *The Prisoner of Sex.* Boston: Little, Brown and Company, 1971.

This book can help females to discover and perhaps understand the tender, vulnerable areas of the apparent male chauvinist. Males can read it and discover that vulnerability is not exclusively their own individual "weakness."

MARTIN, D., LYON, P. *Lesbian Woman.* San Francisco: Glide Publications, 1972. New York: Bantam Edition, 1972.

Extensive, rational, nonmilitant, and nonhysterical information about the pleasures and problems inherent in lesbianism in today's society. The emphasis is on the wide variety of life styles available and practiced, as well as upon the fact that lesbians must consider themselves and be considered by others, first as individuals, second as women, and third as lesbians.

Written by two lesbians who were involved in the organizational phase of the Daughters of Bilitis, now a national lesbian group.

MASTERS, WILLIAM H. and VIRGINIA E. JOHNSON. *Human Sexual Inadequacy.* Boston: Little, Brown and Company, 1970.

See, in particular, for male dysfunction.

———. *Human Sexual Response.* Boston: Little, Brown and Company, 1966.

Superclinical, but the best first-person descriptions of male and female orgasm we have read.

SCHWARZ, RICHARD H. *Septic Abortion.* Philadelphia: J. B. Lippincott Company, 1968.

Primarily for the medical profession. But all of the methods used or considered for self-abortion and the complications of self- and induced abortion are discussed clearly in the first two chapters.

SEGAL, SHELDON. Contraceptive Research: A Male Chauvinist Plot? Family Planning Perspectives, 4: 3 (July) 1972.

SIECUS (Sex Information and Education Council of the United States). SIECUS Study Guides* (50c) 1855 Broadway, New York, New York 10023.

Homosexuality

Masturbation

Characteristics of Male and Female Sexual Responses. (and others, ask for list)

_____. *Sexuality and Man.* New York: Charles Scribner's Sons, 1970.
A compilation of twelve study guides with additional material.

WEST, DONALD J. *Homosexuality.* Rev. ed. Chicago: Aldine Publishing Company, 1968.
Highly recommended, nonjudgmental study of male and female homosexuality. Discusses fundamental research and speculation and clearly identifies areas in which knowledge is still lacking. Also contains a discussion of the historical and contemporary religious and legal aspects of homosexuality.

WYDEN, PETER and BARBARA. *Growing up Straight.** New York: New American Library (Signet Books), 1969.
The only thing judgmental about this book is the title. A paperback that several authorities highly recommend for parents. "What every thoughtful parent should know about homosexuality." Also good for 19- and 20-year-olds.

NOTE: *There are a number of recent publications about male and female homosexuality, some personal accounts, some very general works. It is difficult to recommend any of them without implying that we agree with the particular, almost inevitable, bias that each publication presents, though almost all are enlightening if you are prepared to recognize the bias. The two references on lesbianism are quite rational approaches; we think you can learn from them.*

The exotic "how-to" books, e.g., the "Sensuous" series, are primarily for desperate people. Wait a few years until you are sure that you are desperate or need a change. They could make a number of 20-year-olds feel grossly inadequate. Private tutoring is better than book learning in the area of technique. There are subtle, long-term advantages in allowing your sexuality to evolve spontaneously.

REUBEN, DAVID. *Everything You Always Wanted to Know About Sex but Were Afraid to Ask.** New York: David McKay Company, 1969.

We include this because we made reference to it, and though the underlying philosophy is gentle, the facts, in our area of knowledge, in many cases, are distorted to the point where wrong interpretations may be made upon only a quick reading; and, in many cases the facts are very misleading or in error (a comment also made by many knowledgeable reviewers).

---

* Available in paperback edition.

Acknowledgments

We wish to thank the following people for their help in preparing this book:

Mrs. Alice F. Emerson, Dean of Students, University of Pennsylvania.

Mr. Andrew J. Condon, Dean of Student Activities, University of Pennsylvania.

Members of the Department of Obstetrics and Gynecology at the Hospital of the University of Pennsylvania, especially Drs. Luigi Mastroianni, Jr., Celso-Ramon Garcia, George Povey, and Richard Schwarz.

Dr. Robert Constable, Student Health Service, University of Pennsylvania.

Dr. John Franklin, Department of Obstetrics and Gynecology, Thomas Jefferson University, Philadelphia.

Sidney Callahan, Hastings-on-Hudson, New York, for permission to use her article on chastity.

Dr. Jane Rasmussen (Mrs. Howard R.), Wynnewood, Pennsylvania.

The *Daily Pennsylvanian* for publishing some of these articles and questions and answers, with some modifications, during the 1969-70 school year.

Dr. John Rock, Boston, a special acknowledgment for reading the first edition and offering a number of sophisticated modifications which have been included.

Ellen Cole, Philadelphia, for preparing the original illustrations for the third edition

PLEASE NOTE: *No one of these acknowledgments should be interpreted as any individual's unqualified imprimatur.*

Vulnerable Steps in the Reproductive Process, Male and Female

MALE

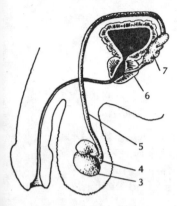

PITUITARY CONTROL (1)

STEROID NEGATIVE FEEDBACK (1 & 2)

SPERM FORMATION IN TESTIS (3)

SPERM MATURATION IN EPIDYDIMIS (4)

SPERM TRANSPORT IN VAS (5)

*SEMINAL FLUID BIOCHEMISTRY
(6 & 7)*

*OVUM TRANSPORT
Ovum pickup by fimbria (5)
Cilia activity (6)
Tubal fluid secretion (6)
Tubal musculature (7)*

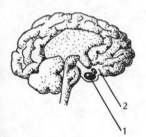

*OVULATION
Steroid negative feedback (1 & 2)
Central nervous system drugs (2)
Gonadotropin antagonists (3)
Local action on follicle (4)*

*ZYGOTE TRANSPORT
Tubal fluid secretion (6)
Tubal musculature (7)*

*FERTILIZATION
Shedding of zona pellucida of ovum (6)
Sperm capacitation (11)
Sperm penetration of egg membrane (6)
Pronuclei fusion (6)*

FEMALE

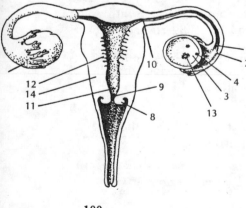

*SPERM TRANSPORT
External os of cervix (8)
Cervical mucus (9)
Utero-tubal junction (10)*

*PREVENTION OF IMPLANTATION
Estrogen binding (12)
Corpus luteum function (13)
Progesterone binding (12)*

*PLACENTATION
Trophoblast formation (12)
Chorionic gonadotropin
production (12)*

*MAINTENANCE OF PREGNANCY
Embryogenesis (12)
Placental function (12)
Myometrial activity (14)*

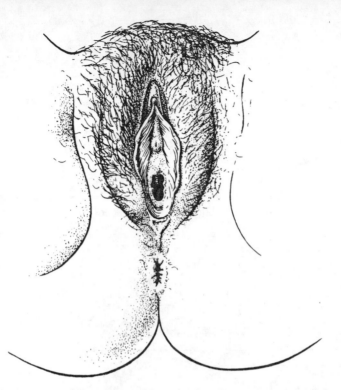

Figure 1. Female perineum, nonvirginal. Labia majora and minora are shown separated. Normally, even with legs spread apart, the labia remain in the midline and the introitus appears closed. The labia minora vary in size, and the relation of the urethral opening to the vagina also varies from one individual to the next. Only the end of the clitoris is ever exposed.

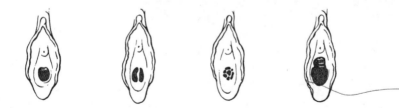

Figure 2. Variations of the hymen. From left to right: virginal, nondilated; septate, septem may or may not stretch; cribiform; parous, at least one full-term delivery. (See Fig. 1 note about introitus.)

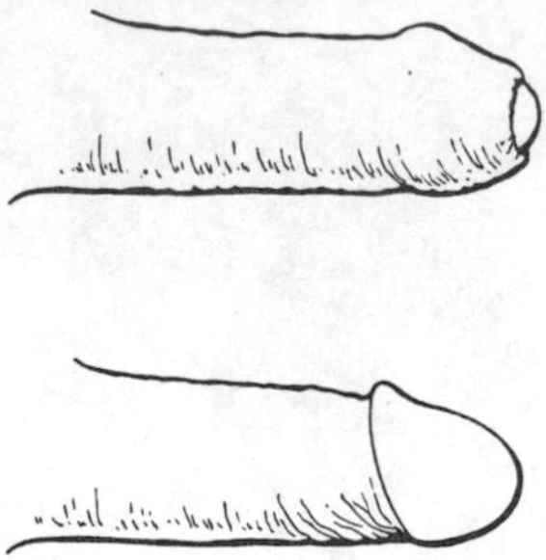

Figure 3. Above: uncircumcised penis, below: circumcised penis. With erection, the foreskin of the former may retract to give the appearance of circumcision. With penetration, the foreskin normally retracts.

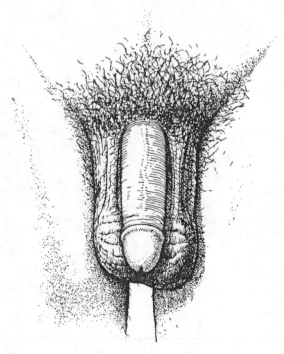

Figure 4. Average adult circumcised male. Note asymmetry of the scrotum and some indication of the spermatic cord. The length of the nonerect penis will vary, as will the size of the scrotum, from one individual to the next. The exaggerated length of the dependent penis in male pornographic magazines is often due to a state of semi-erection.

Index

How many of you have friends who have told you, when they find out that their girl friend is pregnant or that they are pregnant, that it couldn't possibly have happened because . . . . ?

M.

(